the diabetes

D   *gy)*

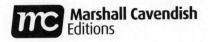
Marshall Cavendish
Editions

Published by Marshall Cavendish Editions
An imprint of Marshall Cavendish International
1 New Industrial Road, Singapore 536196

Other Marshall Cavendish Offices:
Marshall Cavendish International. PO Box 65829 London EC1P 1NY, UK • Marshall Cavendish Corporation. 99 White Plains Road, Tarrytown NY 10591-9001, USA • Marshall Cavendish International (Thailand) Co Ltd. 253 Asoke, 12th Flr, Sukhumvit 21 Road, Klongtoey Nua, Wattana, Bangkok 10110, Thailand • Marshall Cavendish (Malaysia) Sdn Bhd, Times Subang, Lot 46, Subang Hi-Tech Industrial Park, Batu Tiga, 40000 Shah Alam, Selangor Darul Ehsan, Malaysia

Marshall Cavendish is a trademark of Times Publishing Limited

National Library Board, Singapore Cataloguing-in-Publication Data

Lim, Heok Seng.
The diabetes companion / Lim Heok Seng with Jonathan Seah ... [et al.]. – New ed. – Singapore : Marshall Cavendish Editions, 2010.
p. cm.
Includes bibliographical references and index.
ISBN-13 : 978-981-4302-92-0

1. Diabetes – Popular works. I. Title.

RC660.4
616.462 -- dc22   OCN636824231

Printed in Singapore by Times Printers Pte Ltd

CONTENTS

ACKNOWLEDGEMENTS

We would like to record our gratitude to Dr Tavintharan Subramaniam, currently Senior Consultant, Department of Medicine, Alexandra Hospital, and Mrs Joanna Wong, Assistant Director, Clinical Support Services, Changi General Hospital, who were the editors of *Diabetes Totally Uncovered* (a previous in-house publication of Changi General Hospital) which spurred us to write this book.

We very much appreciate the valuable feedback and comments given by Senior Staff Nurses Authilakshmy N Manickam, Sri Rahayu Masjum and Lee Pau Li of the Diabetes Centre, Changi General Hospital.

Thanks also to Dr Emily Ho, Registrar, Department of Endocrinology, Singapore General Hospital, for her valuable comments in the early days of writing this book.

Ms Jessie Phua, Senior Podiatrist, Changi General Hospital, and Mr Jasper Tong, Principal Podiatrist, Podiatry Unit, Singapore General Hospital, were very gracious and prompt in giving useful suggestions on the chapter, 'Foot Problems and Foot Care'.

Ms Ai Ling Sim-Devadas, Assistant Manager, Corporate Affairs, Changi General Hospital, provided much needed administrative support, and was very encouraging throughout the preparation of this book.

We would like also to mention that the staff at the Dietetics and Food Services of Changi General Hospital were very helpful and supportive.

Last but not least, we are thankful to Mr Pradhap Sadasivam and Mr KH Tan, who allowed us to use their actual names/initials for their personal diabetes stories mentioned in Chapter One. To them and to our other patients whose experiences with diabetes we describe in this book, with altered name initials for confidentiality, we are grateful for the many lessons that we have learnt from their experience.

I am very encouraged by the publication of this book which, while simple in format and language, is extremely useful to patients, caregivers and the general public. Written by several key staff of Changi General Hospital, it is backed by decades of experience in managing diabetes in thousands of patients.

Medical science has made great strides in general and for diabetes in particular. Diabetes is a disease on the rise worldwide for the reason that obesity is on the rise. Most patients have Type 2 diabetes because of this. Insulin treatment may not be necessary until the late stage of the disease. So, long before this, there are many treatments and lifestyle changes that can be effectively made to control the disease and prevent complications.

It is my hope that this book will serve its purpose of educating those who need to know about diabetes and its many facets. Knowledge is the essential first step towards better care. It should lead to a change in attitude and lifestyle behaviour. This will result in as near normal a life as possible for the patient.

I congratulate the editor and the authors for this well-written and presented book.

Professor Chee Yam Cheng
Assistant CEO, National Healthcare Group and
Senior Physician, Department of Medicine,
Tan Tock Seng Hospital

"We are here to add what we can to life, not to get what we can from life."

—Sir Dr William Osler (1849–1919)
Canadian-born physician, Father of Modern Medicine

I can safely say that if you are reading this book, either you have diabetes, are at risk of getting it, or know someone (most likely a family member) who has it.

If, indeed, you have diabetes, you have plenty of company. Diabetes is prevalent in epidemic proportions globally. In Singapore, based on the 2004 National Health Survey, 8.2% of adults aged 18 to 69 years (or 328,000 adult residents) have diabetes, half of whom had not been previously diagnosed with the condition in that survey.

It is not surprising, therefore, that hardly a week passes without something being mentioned about diabetes in the local mass media. Some news can be depressing but others hold up hope for diabetics who are waiting for a cure.

Aware of the long-term individual health, social and economic implications of diabetes and its twin problem of obesity, the Ministry of Health, Singapore, is ever looking for more effective ways to prevent and tackle these two conditions head-on.

I have been treating diabetes for the better part of my medical career and am convinced that the role of the person with diabetes, or the person at a high risk of getting diabetes, is crucial. His or her active lifelong participation is integral to the treatment and prevention process. Health authorities, the medical community, and medical science can only do so much, notwithstanding the great advances that have been made in diabetes care in the last 20 years.

Patient education in diabetes self-care gained momentum in the early 1970s, when a landmark study[1] in the United States demonstrated that a group of diabetics who had received diabetes education had fewer hospitalisations, diabetic comas and diabetic foot problems.

It is the responsibility of the health care provider to initiate the education process, but the patient must also be a willing and active partner in order to achieve the best possible therapeutic outcome. He/she must be fully equipped with not only pure or hard facts about the disease, but also the skill to manage it on a day-to-day basis. With diabetes being a 'lifestyle' disease, the patient has to make appropriate choices in the area of diet and physical activity. There are tasks, such as self-monitoring of blood glucose, that he/she must not shy away from.

We have met with many successes where the diabetic person's knowledge, skill and self-motivation contribute significantly to improved health. However, there remains a large number of people with diabetes without a basic knowledge of the condition and how to self-manage it. The reasons are numerous, ranging from failure on the part of the health care professionals and their education programmes to the patients' own lack of interest.

It is, therefore, the objective of this book, *The Diabetes Companion,* to help fill this education gap amongst patients. This book will also serve as a simple reference guide for the medical and health care community interested in the management of diabetes.

The Diabetes Companion is inspired by a previous in-house publication (entitled *Diabetes Totally Uncovered*) which we at the Diabetes Centre in Changi General Hospital were using as a supplement to our personalised diabetes patient self-care, nutrition and foot-care counselling.

This book is different from its predecessor in its style and information. Those familiar with the latter will quickly notice that *The Diabetes Companion* is more detailed, has a more consistent style of presentation, has many updates on treatment guidelines and targets and diabetes medications, and has new chapters, such as 'Interacting with Your Health Care Providers' and 'Alternative Medicines and Supplements'. There are, also, many more real-life anecdotes to illustrate points made in the various sections, and these can be found in the 'List of Cases' page for easy reference. The 'Frequently Asked Questions' section is also larger and consolidated into a separate chapter, to accommodate the numerous questions that patients ask.

In anticipation of a wide and varied readership, I have strived to include something for everyone. Technical jargon has been avoided as much as possible. However, some medical terms are not only unavoidable, but actually add to the understanding of the subject. To explain such terms, I have included a 'Glossary of Medical Jargon'. Terms that are explained as they appear in the text and do not recur elsewhere in the book will not be listed in the glossary.

A list of diabetes resources for further information is provided for readers with further questions.

Each person's diabetes is unique. While the principles of diabetes care spelt out here are applicable to diabetics in general, each individual will have to use the information in consultation with his/her own health care provider within his/her own medical, social and financial context.

As you walk this diabetes journey, we hope you will resolve to continue learning. May *The Diabetes Companion* be your trusted 'buddy', providing the necessary know-how to enable you to be in control of your diabetes, so that you will have a fulfilling life, despite the odds.

"A journey of a thousand miles must begin with a single step."

—*Lao Tzu (604–532 BCE), Chinese philosopher*

Dr Lim Heok Seng
Senior Consultant
Division of Endocrinology, Changi General Hospital
Department of Endocrinology, Singapore General Hospital

HOW TO USE THIS BOOK

At a formal dinner, you are treated first to a cocktail, followed by the appetiser and main course, ending with dessert and coffee (or tea); with good wine flowing throughout the evening. That is the set order of things. You can anticipate what is coming next by the serving sequence.

Although this book is arranged in as orderly and as clinical a fashion as health books ought to be, using it is more like taking a buffet meal. If you prefer, you can take the main course first before the appetiser, and then come back to it again, or go for dessert first, going back and forth as you like. (This is just an analogy. When we are discussing diabetes, we do not want to unwittingly encourage excessive and indiscriminate eating!)

Just like scouring a food menu, you, the reader, can scan the 'Contents' section to 'order' what you like and just enjoy it! The 'List of Cases' page will guide you to real-life diabetes stories (some very inspiring), if that is what you would like to start with first, and it will be like listening to your dining companion or buddy spinning yarn after yarn.

Medical words and terms are listed in the 'Glossary of Medical Jargon'. We suggest that you dip into the glossary as often as necessary and use it as you would, in the same way, consult your dining partner to learn more about the food you are eating. Superscript numbers refer to references in the 'References' chapter at the end of the book.

No matter how you use *The Diabetes Companion*, do remember that it should not and cannot replace any member of your diabetes care team!

INTRODUCTION

YOUR INITIAL REACTION

People discover they have diabetes through many ways—during a pre-employment, annual or pre-national service medical check up, during a health survey, when hospitalised for an unrelated problem, or when symptoms or complications of the disease itself appear.

Whichever it is, it is a rare person who, on being told he has diabetes, would say, "I am just waiting for it." Most would be outright shocked. This shock is all the greater when no one in the family has diabetes and the afflicted has been health-conscious. Some might also go into a period of denial and ignore or delay treatment.

Others would be angry with their parents for passing on the 'diabetic genes' to them. Yet others would be angry that their diabetes was not detected before they developed symptoms or complications. They may also be angry with and blame themselves for overeating and not exercising enough.

Just thinking of the possible complications (heart attack, stroke, kidney failure, eye problems) can bring on anxiety, fear and confusion. It is not surprising, then, that their stress level goes up several notches. Everything around them looks gloomy. Depression can creep in all too easily.

Even those who have had diabetes for a long time get such negative feelings every now and then. This is more so when they have been battling it for a long time at great cost to their physical wellbeing, finances, time, and family and social life.

If you are in this situation, the sooner you accept the diagnosis and not feel angry or sorry for yourself, the easier it is to get your diabetes under control. "Easier said than done," you might say. Your sentiment is quite understandable, but it still has to be said. Of course, it would be nice if your health care providers had said it nicely rather than patronisingly. They probably did not mean to be unkind. Rest assured that they understand what you are going through even if they may say very little and just want to get on with the business of bringing your diabetes under control.

Here's a story to inspire you. To read more on 'Coping with Diabetes and Your Emotions', go to Chapter 14.

Case 1: Mdm YLF – Coming to Terms with Diabetes

Mdm YLF, conscious of the fact that her elder sister had Type 1 diabetes, sought to avert it by reading all about diabetes, eating healthily and exercising regularly. Even when she developed diabetes during her pregnancy while carrying her twins (now six years old), she needed only diet regulation to control her diabetes throughout the pregnancy.

Hence, she was devastated when she developed full-blown diabetes five years later. Her initial three-month average level of blood glucose, measured as glycated haemoglobin (HbA1c), was sky-high at 14.6% (the normal value being 4.5–6.4%). Although it improved to 8.7% with pills, that was the best her GP (general practitioner) could do and she was referred to our Diabetes Centre.

Depression had overtaken her and she had allowed her HbA1c to rise further by not taking her pills for two months. She dared not check her blood sugar, as she could not bear to see high readings, even though she knew they were probably high as she was feeling tired and losing weight.

At the Diabetes Centre, she was duly told that she needed insulin therapy straightaway as she was underweight and her random blood glucose was 22.4 mmol/L (normal being 4–8 mmol/L). Sobbing, Mdm YLF said that she could not accept the fact that, despite her best efforts, she had developed diabetes like her sister. On top of that, she had to undergo frequent gynaecological checkups because of suspicious Pap smear results. She was not comforted by further gynaecologist test results that turned out to be normal.

She denied having excessive urination or thirst, but this was strange as her blood sugar level would definitely have brought about those symptoms.

Linking her present diabetes to her first encounter with diabetes during pregnancy, she expressed her anger at her children.

She apologised to her doctor for breaking down, saying that diabetes may be something that doctors thought nothing of (as they see it everyday) but it was a really big blow to her. She was worried that she might need insulin for life.

She even planned to quit her job as the company she worked in was in the process of being taken over and there was "too much company politics". Everything bad appeared worse.

To the doctor's relief, after the protracted ventilation, she agreed to start insulin therapy. Three weeks later, she was all smiles. Injecting her insulin as prescribed had lowered her self-monitored blood sugar to between 4.6 and 11.2 mmol/L. Not a word of despair, no gripes, and the consultation was over in 15 minutes.

Comments: Mdm YLF turned out to have Latent Autoimmune Diabetes of Adult (LADA), a form of diabetes that has features of both Type 1 and Type 2 diabetes (see Chapter 2).

Case 2: Mdm HJG – "Little Drops of Water..."

Mdm HJG, a 58-year-old Type 2 diabetic, had poor diabetes control for some time. She also had high blood pressure and cataract, and had laser treatment for diabetic eye disease. Her usual meal routine was two big meals a day and she was "too lazy" to exercise.

One day, she surprised her doctor when her HbA1c improved modestly from 9.1% to 8.1% (the ideal for her was 7% or less). It turned out that she had finally made the following changes: having three smaller meals daily instead of two big meals, eating less rice and fried fish (her favourite) but more vegetables, and doing light callisthenic exercises every morning before going to work. The improvement in blood sugar control was all the 'sweeter' as she had also stopped taking one of the diabetes pills which she believed was causing her legs to swell. She was beaming with pride as she related her changed lifestyle. Her HbA1c improved further to 7.1% three months later.

Case 2 was inspired by another patient who admitted to his doctor that he had been skipping his diabetes pill and hardly exercised. When urged to remember to take his medicine regularly, he asked sceptically, "Does it really make a difference?" Every little effort certainly counts!

"Little drops of water, little grains of sand,
make the mighty ocean and the beauteous land."

—*Robert Louis Stevenson (1850–1894)*
Scottish novelist, essayist and poet

Remember, every little effort counts. The case of Mdm HJG illustrates this point.

There are many more stories in this book. However, for now, it is important that you know:

THE ESSENTIALS OF MANAGING YOUR DIABETES

- Accept it, have a positive attitude, and move on.
- Do as much for yourself as you can.
- Know as much about diabetes as possible and separate myth from truth.
- Understand that a suitable diet and exercise (if not medically contraindicated) are necessary for life.
- Maintain a healthy weight.
- Take your medications as prescribed.
- Monitor your blood sugar.
- Go for regular check-ups.
- Watch out for complications of diabetes and get early treatment.
- Have an open and proper interaction with your health care providers.
- Develop a healthy optimism.

01 UNDERSTANDING DIABETES MELLITUS—
The Basics

"To understand is hard. Once one understands, action is easy."

—Dr Sun Yat-sen (1866–1925)
Chinese revolutionary and Father of Modern China

Diabetes mellitus has been around for centuries. It has to be differentiated from the much rarer condition called 'diabetes insipidus', which has the common symptom of increased urination but has nothing to do with blood glucose or sugar. Throughout this book, the word 'diabetes' will be used to refer to diabetes mellitus. The words 'sugar' and 'glucose' will be used synonymously unless otherwise stated.

Diabetes is a condition in which the body is unable to maintain blood glucose within the normal physiological range, due to either an inadequate production of insulin or ineffective insulin action, or both. The hallmark of diabetes is, therefore, high blood glucose or hyperglycaemia.

WHAT NORMALLY HAPPENS IN YOUR BODY (Fig 1)
Let us first understand where sugar comes from and how our body handles it. Sugar comes not just from sweetened foods (like candy and regular soft drinks) but also from non-sweet complex carbohydrate foods, such as rice, bread, potatoes, pasta, noodles, *chapatti*, *naan*, and some vegetables (like carrots). It is important to correct the common misunderstanding that as long as a food does not taste sweet, it does not contribute to the sugar in the bloodstream. It will, if it contains absorbable carbohydrates, sweet or otherwise!

Glucose or sugar per se is not evil. In fact, it is an essential nutrient to all our tissues and organs. It is the primary source of energy, much like petrol provides the energy needed to move a car. Blood sugar levels are closely controlled by hormones. The main and most important of these hormones is insulin, which is produced by specialised cells, called beta-cells, in the islets of Langerhans in the pancreas. Another hormone, glucagon, produced by the alpha-cells, also in the islets of Langerhans, plays a secondary role. The rise in blood sugar after a meal stimulates the release of insulin and suppresses that of glucagon.

Insulin binds with insulin receptors on cells of organs and tissues, enabling the sugar to get inside. The action is like that of keys (insulin) fitting into keyholes (insulin receptors), unlocking the cell 'doors' to let the sugar in. Inside the cells, glucose is used for energy production to maintain the function of the body. Any excess glucose, not immediately needed for energy production, is stored in the muscles and liver as storage glucose or glycogen.

The liver plays a vital role in blood sugar regulation under the influence of insulin and glucagon. It has the capacity to make sugar by breaking down glycogen, as well as synthesising it from proteins and releasing it into the blood. After a meal, the high insulin level dampens this effect. Hours after a meal, as well as overnight, when the sugar level has dropped, insulin release is automatically reduced or switched off, and the liver starts to make and release sugar by the action of glucagon, which now kicks into action. In this way, the blood sugar is always kept tightly within a normal physiological range.

WHAT HAPPENS IN DIABETES (Fig 2, 3)

In diabetes, either there are not enough of these 'keys', or the 'keyholes' are not enough or faulty. That is to say, there is either insufficient insulin or the insulin is not able to carry out its function because of insufficient or inefficient insulin receptors, a condition called insulin resistance. As a result, sugar builds up in the blood.

As the cells are not getting the sugar, stored fats are broken down into fatty acids, which are then used as an alternative energy source to maintain function and life of the organ or tissue. These fatty acids are released into the bloodstream and transported to the liver, where they are converted to ketones. Large amounts of ketones make the blood acidic and are potentially dangerous (see Chapter 2).

Another effect of insulin resistance is that the liver will continue to make and release sugar into the bloodstream, even when there is still plenty of sugar, thus raising the blood sugar further.

When blood sugar reaches a critical level, it will be filtered by the kidneys into the urine and, hence, the urine will be loaded with glucose (glycosuria). Filtered sugar carries along with it lots of free water and this is why the diabetic person passes more urine. A lot of water is thus lost from the body, which then senses that it is dehydrated, and the person will start to drink lots of fluid. If he does not yet know he has diabetes, he will usually go for sugary fluids because his body actually senses that he does not have enough energy, since the sugar is not getting into the cells, but merely staying in the bloodstream. He is actually 'starving in the presence of plenty'. Drinking sugary fluids will, of course, raise the blood sugar further. He feels progressively tired and loses weight as more and more fat (as well as protein) is being used to provide alternative energy.

Figure 1. How our body maintains normal blood glucose

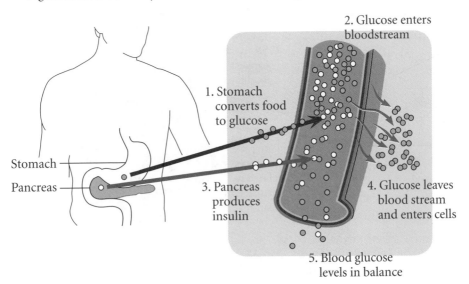

2. Glucose enters bloodstream

1. Stomach converts food to glucose

Stomach

Pancreas

3. Pancreas produces insulin

4. Glucose leaves blood stream and enters cells

5. Blood glucose levels in balance

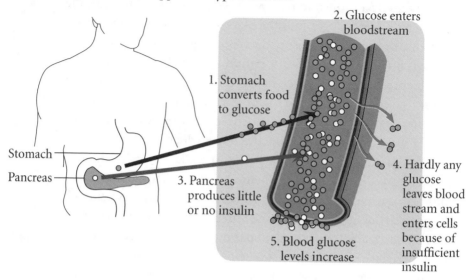

Figure 2. What happens in Type 1 diabetes

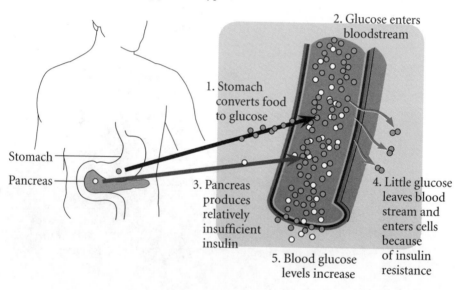

Figure 3. What happens in Type 2 diabetes

SYMPTOMS OF DIABETES

Diabetes, in its early stages, may not give rise to any symptoms and is, thus, often first diagnosed only during routine blood tests. In more severe stages, the classic symptoms of diabetes are as follows:

- Increased urination
- Excessive thirst
- Increased hunger
- Weight loss despite a normal or even good appetite
- General tiredness and weakness
- Nausea and vomiting (only in severe diabetes)

You may also be alerted to possible diabetes if you notice:
- Ants attracted to your urine
- Positive urine sugar test*
- Blurred vision (because of too much sugar in the eye lens)
- Recurrent skin infection (because high blood sugar is a risk for infection)
- Slow healing of cuts and wounds
- Numbness of the feet
- Any symptoms related to any of the chronic diabetic complications (see Chapter 2).

*In the past, diabetes was solely recognised by the presence of sugar in the urine and, hence, in many vernacular languages, the disease is literally described as 'sugary urine sickness' (*tang niao bing* in Chinese) or 'sweet urine' (*kencing manis* in Malay).

WHO GETS DIABETES?

Diabetes affects people of all age groups and races. In Singapore, about 8.2% of adults (aged 18 to 69 years) have diabetes, and its prevalence increases with age. More than 90% of diabetics are over 40 years old. Amongst the three main ethnic groups in Singapore, the Indians have the highest prevalence, followed by the Malays, then the Chinese.

A person is at high risk of getting diabetes if he has any of the risk factors listed below. The level of risk corresponds with the number of risk factors:
- Family history of diabetes
- Overweight and obese
- Sedentary lifestyle
- Above 40 years old
- Pregnancy

- High blood pressure (hypertension)
- Abnormal lipid (fat) levels (high triglyceride and low HDL-cholesterol)
- History of gestational diabetes mellitus (see below)
- Pre-diabetes (see below)
- HbA1c between 5.7 and 6.4% (marker of average blood glucose over 2–3 months)
- Clinical conditions associated with insulin resistance, such as polycystic ovarian syndrome.

TYPES OF DIABETES

Although diabetes is characterised by high blood glucose, it is not a single specific disease but is actually quite heterogeneous, with different causes. The various types of diabetes are classified as follows:

1. Type 1 Diabetes (Figure 2)

Type 1 diabetes is less common than Type 2 diabetes. In Type 1 diabetes, the patient produces little or no insulin. It is caused by an altered immune system (the system that produces antibodies to fight off foreign invaders, such as bacteria and viruses) which mistakenly destroys the insulin producing cells in the pancreas. Hence, Type 1 diabetes is considered an autoimmune disease ('auto' means 'self' and 'autoimmune' implies immune reaction against self). The insulin deficiency in Type 1 diabetes is so severe that insulin is needed as soon as the diagnosis is made. It usually develops in children and young adults, but no age group is spared, although it is rarely seen in the elderly. Type 1 diabetes is always accompanied by symptoms and may even present with ketoacidosis (see Chapter 2).

Case 3: Mr Pradhap Sadasivan – Personal Account of Type 1 Diabetes

"I was first diagnosed with Type 1 diabetes in November 1996 while I was working in Pittsburgh, USA. I was 30 years old then. Prior to the diagnosis, I experienced severe thirst, frequent urination and weight loss of 15 kg. In December 1996, I returned to Singapore to seek treatment, where I was placed on insulin injections (three regular short-acting insulin injections daily before each meal and a single intermediate-acting insulin injection at bedtime). With strong support from my wife, who is a trained cytotechnologist, I embarked on a programme of balanced diet, regular exercise and regular blood glucose monitoring before and two hours after meals. Because of my strong family history of diabetes, hypertension and heart disease, I decided to revamp my carefree lifestyle.

Sometime in 2005, I was diagnosed with hypertension as well as hypothyroidism (low thyroid hormone), which my doctor said was associated with Type 1 diabetes. I was experiencing the following symptoms: bulging varicose veins in my legs; lack of sweating after vigorous exercise; and lethargy, despite having sufficient hours of sleep.

I am now using the 24-hour action insulin glargine with three shots of rapid-acting insulin aspart before my meals. I continue to see my doctor once every six months. About two to three hours before the consultation, blood samples are taken to determine my lipid (fats) profile, sugar profile and thyroid function. I am happy that recent results showed that my total cholesterol was 120 mg/dL (3.07 mmol/L), fasting glucose 110 mg/dL (6.1 mmol/L) and HbA1c 6.7%, which my doctor said reflected good control. My thyroid function tests were also normal. Once a year, I go through a complete screening for eye, foot and kidney complications. I do not have any of these so far. I do get the occasional hypoglycaemia (low blood glucose) episodes, typically when my lunch is delayed, but they are mild. I am still doing my best to balance my meals, activity and insulin."

2. Type 2 Diabetes (Figure 3)

About 90% of people with diabetes have Type 2 diabetes. If you have Type 2 diabetes, you have come through a stage called 'pre-diabetes' of variable duration (see box below).

As an extension of, and like, pre-diabetes, Type 2 diabetes is characterised by insulin resistance. Type 2 diabetic people can still produce insulin but the amount produced is not enough to overcome the insulin resistance. Ironically, they may even produce more insulin than a non-diabetic person in the early phase of the disease in an effort to overcome the insulin resistance. A major cause of insulin resistance is obesity.

Type 2 diabetes is usually controlled, initially, by diet and exercise with or without oral medications. Insulin is usually not required, but may become necessary as the condition progresses. If, at the time of diagnosis, however, the blood sugar is very high and the patient has symptoms, insulin may be required.

Pre-diabetes

Pre-diabetes is not a condition you can feel, as it does not cause symptoms. There is evidence that at this 'very early' stage, there is insulin resistance and, although diabetes has not yet developed, there is already a higher risk of heart disease and stroke. There are two subsets of pre-diabetes called Impaired Glucose Tolerance (IGT) and Impaired Fasting Glucose (IFG).

In Singapore, the prevalence of IGT is 12%. People with IGT are more likely to develop diabetes compared to those without it. Regular exercise and prudent diet and weight reduction in those who are overweight have all been shown to be effective in preventing this phase from worsening to frank diabetes. Although several drugs have similar benefits, their use for this purpose is still not widely practised, except in those with many other risk factors for developing diabetes.

Case 4: Mr KH Tan – Facing up to Type 2 Diabetes

Mr KH Tan is a 58-year-old businessman who had bypass surgery for coronary heart disease when he was 56. In February 2008, he started to experience thirst which he would satisfy by drinking lots of sugarcane water, although he never enjoyed sweet (or salty) food and drinks before. He was also passing more urine. In three weeks, he lost 10 kg. He was happy to lose weight, but his wife sensed that something was wrong.

When Mr Tan went for his routine exercise at the Heart Wellness Centre at Bishan Junction 8, his wife confided in the physiotherapist there. The physiotherapist checked his blood glucose and found it to be very high (around 23 mmol/L). She quickly stopped Mr Tan from exercising further and got him to see a doctor at the same shopping mall. The doctor confirmed that his glucose was indeed very high and prescribed him a week's medicine with the advice to consult his heart doctor at the National Heart Centre as soon as possible.

Mr Tan was initially very scared and refused to believe that he had diabetes because nobody in his family had it. He even did a test "the traditional way" (his own words) by leaving his urine on a spot where there were ants, to see if the ants would be attracted to it. They were not. (This was rather unusual given the extremely high level of his blood glucose. Mr Tan joked that perhaps the ants were already well-fed.)

Later, when his heart doctor confirmed his diabetes, he still did not believe it. It took further explanations by his doctor before he accepted it and took the prescribed medications, tolbutamide and metformin, and saw the dietitian for advice on a suitable diet.

Finally convinced that he had diabetes and that, with a proper diet, his glucose level could be controlled, Mr Tan started to check his blood sugar regularly with a glucose meter. After 10 days of treatment, his glucose level went back to normal and all his symptoms disappeared.

Mr Tan has this to say about diabetes: it is "no joking matter", and he advises people with diabetes to follow the dietitian's advice on food. His latest HbA1c was 6.8% compared to 12.3% initially.

Table 1: Major differences between Type 1 and Type 2 diabetes

Type 1 Diabetes	Type 2 Diabetes
No or very little insulin reserve	Insulin reserve available, but its actions are compromised by insulin resistance
Usually occurs in those below 30 years old	Usually occurs in those above 40 years old, with a strong family history of diabetes
Affected person is usually lean	Affected person is often overweight
Always exhibits acute symptoms; prone to ketoacidosis	May or may not have symptoms

Diabetes, genes and the environment
Both Type 1 and Type 2 diabetes are the result of complex multiple genetic defects interacting with environmental factors. Obesity and sedentary lifestyle are strongly linked to Type 2 diabetes, as mentioned earlier, while certain viruses are believed to be associated with Type 1 diabetes. These genetic and trigger factors are not fully understood.

Atypical Diabetes
Most people with diabetes can be classified as having either Type 1 or Type 2 diabetes, although there is a minority which cannot be easily classified because they exhibit some features of both types of diabetes. While research continues to understand and define these different subtypes, at present, they are arbitrarily labelled as 'atypical diabetes'.

An example is Latent Autoimmune Diabetes in Adults (LADA) (refer to the case of Mdm YLF in the 'Introduction' chapter). Although it is caused by autoimmunity (like Type 1 diabetes), it develops in relatively older people (like Type 2 diabetes). The initial insulin deficiency is not so severe as to require insulin, but its dependence on insulin soon shows up.

Another example, called Flatbush diabetes, is closer to Type 2 diabetes in many aspects, but people who have it are more prone to diabetic ketoacidosis (like Type 1 diabetes).

This illustrates that diabetes is not a single disease, hence your doctor may have to run several tests to better understand which type of diabetes you have.

3. Gestational Diabetes Mellitus (GDM)

This form of diabetes occurs during pregnancy in women without a previous history of diabetes. Women who have a family history of diabetes and who are obese are more prone to develop GDM. It usually resolves after childbirth, but may reappear in subsequent pregnancies. In some women, the diabetes persists after childbirth and, depending on a number of clinical and biochemical features, they will be classified as having Type 1 or Type 2 diabetes.

4. Other Specific Types of Diabetes

A final grouping of diabetes contains a long list of clinical syndromes and diseases in which diabetes is a component feature or occurs as an association. It includes many congenital syndromes, congenital rubella infection and a condition called maturity-onset diabetes of the young (MODY); the latter is due to a defect in a single gene that affects the production of insulin. Others in this mixed bag are specific diseases of the pancreas, such as chronic pancreatitis (inflammation of the pancreas), surgical removal of the pancreas and pancreas tumour, due to loss of insulin-producing cells in these conditions. Diseases that cause overproduction of thyroid hormones (hyperthyroidism), growth hormones and adrenal hormones can also cause diabetes because these hormones oppose the action of insulin. Steroid drugs used for conditions such as asthma and rheumatoid arthritis can also lead to diabetes because these drugs oppose the action of insulin.

DIAGNOSING DIABETES AND PRE-DIABETES

Although the presence of sugar in the urine is common in diabetes, the diagnosis is strictly based on *blood* glucose level.

In the presence of typical symptoms, the diagnosis of diabetes can be made when either:

1. Fasting blood glucose is 7 mmol/L or higher, or
2. Random blood glucose is 11.1 mmol/L or higher.

Without symptoms, either of the above readings must be obtained on more than one occasion for the diagnosis to be confirmed, unless they are clearly well above the cut-off levels.

The American Diabetes Association has recently recommended that an HbA1c greater than 6.5% is also diagnostic of diabetes, provided the HbA1c test is done in an appropriate laboratory.

Impaired Fasting Glucose (IFG) is diagnosed if the fasting blood glucose is between 5.6 and 6.9 mmol/L and blood glucose two hours after ingesting 75 g of glucose is below 7.8 mmol/L in an Oral Glucose Tolerance Test (OGTT).

Impaired Glucose Tolerance (IGT) is present when the fasting blood glucose is less than 7.0 mmol/L and the blood glucose two hours after ingesting 75 g of glucose is between 7.8 and 11.1 mmol/L in the OGTT.

Note: The above values are seemingly odd because they are in SI units (Système International d'Unités or International System of Units) and are conversions from the rounded non-SI units still used in the USA. To convert blood glucose values in SI units to non-SI units, multiply by 18. Hence, 7.0 mmol/L = 126 mg/dL, 7.8 mmol/L = 140 mg/dL and 11.1 mmol/L = 200 mg/dL.

THE TOTALITY OF DIABETES

Although pre-diabetes and diabetes are strictly defined by blood glucose levels and we have been focusing on blood sugar, they are often closely associated with obesity, high blood pressure and an abnormal lipid (fats) profile. It cannot be over-emphasized that, apart from blood glucose, all these associated problems must be controlled to give you the best chance of keeping at bay the symptoms and complications of the disease.

02 COMPLICATIONS OF DIABETES

"The strongest oak tree of the forest is not the one that is protected from the storm and hidden from the sun. It's the one that stands in the open where it is compelled to struggle for its existence against the winds and rains and the scorching sun."

—Dr Napoleon Hill (1883–1970)
American author and motivational speaker

Diabetes is a serious disease because of the potential complications. In medical language, a complication of a disease is simply a condition that arises if the primary disease is not adequately treated or controlled. Thus, we speak of heart failure being a complication of uncontrolled hypertension (high blood pressure) and stomach bleeding a potential complication of untreated stomach ulcer.

The sad truth about diabetes is that its complications can affect almost any organ in the body and also many organs simultaneously, as they are all awash with sugar, fats and subjected to blood pressure. Some of these complications occur within a short time, while others develop slowly over a longer time without obvious symptoms until something dramatic, like a heart attack, strikes. Hence diabetes is often dubbed "the silent killer".

Diabetic complications are, therefore, conveniently classified as either acute or chronic complications.

ACUTE DIABETIC COMPLICATIONS
Acute complications develop over a short period of time, sometimes quite suddenly:

Diabetic Ketoacidosis (DKA)

In diabetic ketoacidosis, the blood sugar may rise to as high as 20–40 mmol/L (the normal range being 4–8 mmol/L). The signs and symptoms are extreme thirst, increased urination, abdominal pain, vomiting, breathlessness, dehydration, low blood pressure, drowsiness and even coma. In this condition, because sugar is not getting into the cells and tissues, large amounts of fats are broken down or 'burnt' to provide alternative energy. This produces lots of organic acid (called ketones) in the blood (hence 'ketoacidosis'). The respiratory system goes into overdrive in an attempt to blow out the carbon dioxide generated by the acidosis, and the patient finds himself breathing deeply and rapidly, giving the sensation of breathlessness. Not uncommonly, DKA may be the first manifestation of Type 1 diabetes. DKA can also occur in pre-existing Type 1 or Type 2 diabetes when control has been severely compromised by failure to maintain proper treatment or by a precipitating stressful event like infection, a heart attack or injury. It is a medical emergency that can only be adequately treated in the hospital to prevent a fatal outcome.

Hyperosmolar Hyperglycaemia Syndrome (HHS)

In hyperosmolar hyperglycaemia syndrome, the blood sugar is also very high and may reach 50–60 mmol/L over a few days. There is severe dehydration causing low blood pressure. Confusion and coma may occur rapidly as a result of very concentrated blood caused by the very high sugar content. However, the blood is not acidic and the patient, who is usually an elderly Type 2 diabetic, does not usually feel breathless. Like DKA, it is often precipitated by other severe physical illnesses or injuries, and also by inadequate fluid intake. It is also a medical emergency with a very high mortality rate, if it is not quickly and adequately treated.

Hypoglycaemia (Low Blood Glucose or Sugar)

Strictly speaking, hypoglycaemia is not a complication of diabetes itself, but a complication of diabetes treatment. This is because the current methods we use to treat diabetes are, unfortunately, not perfect as they are attempts to balance the effects of medications with food intake and physical activity. If the medication is more than you need for the moment, or if you eat less or exercise more, blood sugar can drop to below normal. We consider it a complication of diabetes because the problem can be traced to the fact that in diabetes, your pancreas is not able to regulate the blood sugar levels. Because hypoglycaemia is such an important topic, we have devoted a whole chapter to it (see Chapter 6).

Infections

Poorly controlled diabetes increases the risk of infections. This is because the white blood cells that normally counter infection do not function very well when the blood sugar is chronically high. Urinary tract infection (UTI) is particularly common in women, especially when there is urine retention caused by a weak bladder from neuropathy (see below). The retained urine is a rich pool for bacteria growth. The symptoms of UTI, if present, are frequent and painful urination and fever. Other common infections are pneumonia, gall bladder infection, skin infection and vaginal yeast infection. An overwhelming infection causes septicaemia, commonly called blood poisoning, when it spreads into the blood. Although infections usually clear up with antibiotic drugs, it is better to avoid having them by paying meticulous attention to diabetes control and personal hygiene.

CHRONIC DIABETIC COMPLICATIONS

Chronic diabetic complications generally take years to appear.

Heart and Blood Vessel Diseases (Cardiovascular Disease or CVD)

The triad of cardiovascular disease are:

1. Coronary artery disease or CAD (which causes heart attack)
2. Cerebral thrombosis (which causes stroke)
3. Peripheral vascular disease or PVD (which causes pain and gangrene in the lower limbs)

These conditions are caused by poor blood supply due to a combination of factors, including cholesterol plaques on the inner wall of blood vessels, inflammatory reactions to these deposits, tendency for the blood to clot, and destructive free radicals. The risk of CVD is further increased by high blood pressure, smoking and an unhealthy lipid profile (see Table 2).

Table 2: Unhealthy lipid profile

LDL- cholesterol ('bad' cholesterol)	Above 2.5 mmol/L
HDL- cholesterol ('good' cholesterol)	Below 1.0 mmol/L
Triglyceride	Above 1.6 mmol/L

Diabetes increases the risk of heart attack by two to four times and heart disease is the major cause of death in the elderly diabetic. A typical heart attack causes chest pain, breathlessness and sweating. Diabetics may sometimes not feel any pain during a heart attack because of cardiac neuropathy (see below). In this situation, the first indication would be breathlessness, low blood pressure or abnormal heart rhythm.

Diabetes increases the risk of a stroke by five times. A stroke usually, but not always, manifests as weakness or paralysis of the arm and leg on one side of the body. The presentation depends on which cerebral blood vessel is blocked and which part of the brain is deprived of adequate blood supply.

PVD typically presents itself with pain in the feet or legs, initially only during walking and later even at rest. The toes might feel cold and wounds do not heal easily, causing gangrene. In Singapore, an estimated 700 lower limb amputations related to diabetic PVD are carried out each year.

Diabetic Eye Diseases

Diabetes is the most common cause of blindness in developed countries. People with diabetes are four times more likely to go blind than those without it. Diabetic eye diseases include cataracts, glaucoma and retinal diseases (diabetic retinopathy). The retina is the light-sensitive innermost lining of the eyeball. After15 years of diabetes, 80% of diabetics show some signs of retinopathy. For more on this subject, see Chapter 8.

Kidney Disease (Diabetic Nephropathy)

Nephropathy is a general term referring to kidney damage or disease. When it is due to diabetes, it is called diabetic nephropathy. It is the result of longstanding poor diabetes control, aggravated by high blood pressure and smoking, and can lead to gradual kidney failure. In its earliest stage, small amounts of albumin, a type of protein, appears in the urine because the filtering membranes of the kidneys are leaky and not able to hold it back. This is the stage of microalbuminuria. If the condition is not arrested, more and more albumin will appear in the urine (stage of macroalbuminuria). Timely detection of albumin in the urine is therefore vital to detect the condition and to initiate aggressive preventive measures.

Nerve Disease (Diabetic Neuropathy)

Neuropathy is a general term referring to nerve damage and dysfunction due to many different causes. When it is due to diabetes, it is called diabetic neuropathy. Like the other complications of diabetes mentioned above, diabetic neuropathy is also the result of longstanding poor diabetes control. Since every part and organ of our body is supplied by nerves, diabetic neuropathy can cause widespread multi-organ malfunction.

Peripheral Neuropathy

In peripheral neuropathy, nerves in the legs and feet malfunction. The earliest symptom is numbness and tingling in the toes and feet. With time, loss of sensation sets in and there is the risk of injuring your feet without feeling or knowing about the injury unless you make a conscious effort to look for signs of injury. Infection may set in, especially if blood sugar is high, and there is also poor blood supply from PVD. Gangrene and amputations are then potential threats. For more on this, see Chapter 9.

Sometimes, the nerve damage in the legs do not produce the symptoms described above, but instead causes progressive weakness and wasting of the leg muscles.

Then again, the nerve malfunction may affect a single muscle and causes localised paralysis, such as paralysis of eye muscles leading to double vision.

Autonomic Neuropathy

The autonomic nervous system is the network of nerves that controls and regulates the function of the various internal organs, such as the heart, lungs, stomach, etc. Autonomic neuropathy or malfunctioning of autonomic nerves can cause a host of signs and symptoms that include:

- Stomach bloating due to slow emptying of the stomach
- Diarrhoea or constipation
- Urination difficulty and urine retention due to a weak bladder contraction
- Gallstone formation due to retention of bile in the gallbladder
- Sexual impotence due to loss of nerve function (as well as poor blood flow) in the genital organ
- Silent heart attack, postural hypotension (excessive drop in blood pressure on rising from a sitting or lying position), and poor cardiac response to exercise due to cardiac nerve dysfunction (cardiac neuropathy)
- Poor temperature regulation
- Reduced thirst sensation

Prevention and Treatment

Many of these chronic diabetic complications do not have effective treatment and the best approach is prevention. As the saying goes, "a stitch in time saves nine." Therefore, take your diabetes seriously. It is mostly about controlling your blood sugar, blood pressure and lipids, not smoking, early detection and personal vigilance.

Specific medicines to reduce the tendency of the blood to clot, such as aspirin, ticlodipine and clopidogrel, are indicated for those at high risk of blood vessel blockage and those who are already showing signs of blockage. Bypass grafting surgery, angioplasty or ballooning, or insertion of stents may be required to overcome the blood vessel blockage.

In early diabetic nephropathy, when significant amounts of albumin appear in the urine, a number of drugs can be used to prevent the condition from worsening. These are members of two groups of drugs called Angiotensin Converting Enzyme Inhibitors (ACE inhibitors) and Angiotensin Receptor Blockers (ARB). When terminal kidney failure occurs, dialysis or kidney transplantation is the only solution.

Diabetic neuropathy is difficult to treat and treatment is usually only to relieve symptoms. The treatment available for diabetic eye diseases is briefly discussed in Chapter 8.

Landmark Studies on Blood Glucose Control and Complications

- The Diabetes Control and Complications Trial (DCCT)[1], showed that in Type 1 diabetes, maintaining near normal blood sugar can reduce the risk of eye disease by 76%, kidney disease by 50%, and nerve damage by 60%.
- The United Kingdom Prospective Diabetes Study (UKPDS)[2] showed that in Type 2 diabetics, treatment aimed at achieving near normal blood sugar resulted in a 25% reduction of combined retinal, kidney and nerve complications, as well as a suggestion, albeit weaker, that the risk of cardiovascular complications was also reduced.

The downside of intensive therapy to normalise blood sugar control in these studies was greater weight gain and more frequent severe hypoglycaemia. Although this therefore makes intensive therapy unsuitable for some patients, near normal blood sugar control should be the goal for the majority.

In a follow-up study to the DCCT, the Epidemiology of Diabetes Interventions and Complications (EDIC) study[3] showed that even when well controlled patients subsequently slipped up in their blood sugar control, they had fewer complications than those who had higher blood sugar initially. Conversely, those who had poor control initially but did better later, still had more complications. The inference is that near normal sugar control should be achieved as early as possible.

Keeping diabetic complications away—an eight-point plan

1. Keep your blood sugar, blood pressure and lipid profile as normal as possible
2. Exercise regularly
3. Do not smoke
4. Maintain an ideal body weight
5. Recognise the symptoms and seek early treatment
6. Go for regular screening for early detection of complications
7. Consult your diabetes care team regularly
8. Take appropriate medications for specific complications

Case 5: Mr KM - Keeping Complications at Bay

Mr KM is a 53-year-old diabetic who was doing fairly well with an HbA1c of 7.5%. This was not perfect but better than most. He had, in the past, a near perfect score of 6.9%. Then, for six months in 2006, he lost control and saw his HbA1c rising to 9%. He was frank enough to admit that he had not been taking his medications regularly. He would sometimes skip them for one whole week when overseas, or would not take them for a few days after he had taken alcohol in the evening. At 79 kg and with a BMI of 26.7 kg/m², he was clinically obese. He made renewed efforts to straighten things out and even joined the weight management programme at the Changi Sports Medicine Centre of Changi General Hospital. After a month, he shed 1 kg. He cut down his drinking and took his medications regularly. His HbA1c dropped to 7.6%. This improvement, if sustained, will effectively reduce his risk of chronic complications by more than 40%.

03 TREATING DIABETES

PART 1: TACKLING OBESITY

*"The pessimist finds difficulty in every opportunity;
the optimist finds opportunity in every difficulty."*

—Lawrence Pearsall Jacks (1860–1955)
English writer, educator and philosopher

If you are overweight with pre-diabetes or Type 2 diabetes, you would do well to shed some of those extra fats for better control of your blood sugar, blood pressure and fat levels, apart from reducing your risk of getting the complications listed in Table 3.

Table 3: Medical conditions associated with obesity

Diabetes and pre-diabetes
High blood pressure
Coronary heart disease
High triglycerides and low HDL-cholesterol
Obstructive sleep apnoea
Back and knee problems
Gallstones
Cancers: colorectal, liver, stomach, kidney, prostate, breast, uterus and ovaries
Infertility in women
Varicose veins
Depression

This chapter provides general principles on weight reduction. More details on diet and exercise can be found in the next two chapters.

WHAT IS OBESITY?

Obesity is defined as the accumulation of excessive body fat to the extent that it may cause or has caused health problems. You can be overweight and yet have healthy amounts of fat if your bone structure and lean body mass (muscles) are large. An example is body builders in whom muscles contribute relatively more to body weight than fats. At the other end of the spectrum, an elderly person can have a normal weight for his height and yet have increased body fat relative to his lean body mass. In this book, the words 'overweight' and 'obesity' are used synonymously to mean excessive unhealthy accumulation of body fat.

MEASURING OBESITY

There are many ways to measure obesity. In clinical practice, two practical ways of measuring obesity are:

Body Mass Index (BMI)

This is a simple indicator of whether you are overweight or not. It is calculated by dividing one's body weight in kilograms by the square of one's height in metres.

$$\text{Body mass index} = \frac{\text{Weight (kg)}}{\text{Height (m) x Height (m)}}$$

What is a healthy BMI? In this respect, Asians and Caucasians differ slightly. For Caucasians, a BMI between 18.5 kg/m² and 24.9 kg/m² is considered ideal but for Asians it is 18.5 kg/m² to 22.9 kg/m². This is because for the same BMI, the average Asian has more body fat than the average Caucasian and, therefore, a higher cardiovascular risk.

The risk of cardiovascular disease and diabetes is greater the higher the BMI as shown in Table 4:

Table 4: BMI and the risk of heart disease and diabetes[1]

BMI (kg/m^2) (for adults)	Risk of Heart Disease and Diabetes, etc.
35 and above	Very high risk
27.5 and above	High risk
23.0–27.4	Moderate risk
18.5–22.9	Low risk (healthy range)
Less than 18.5	Risk of nutritional deficiency diseases and osteoporosis

Note: MOH Clinical Practice Guidelines 5/2004-Obesity.

Type 2 diabetes is ten times more common in those with a body mass index of 27–30 kg/m^2. It is not uncommon to see Type 2 diabetics with a BMI above 30 kg/m^2.

Waist Circumference and Waist-to-Hip Ratio

The BMI may not always be an accurate measure of body fat as some people may have a high BMI because of larger muscle and bone structure rather than fat. Moreover, it is the amount of fat inside the abdomen (central obesity) that is associated with coronary heart disease. The waist circumference and waist-to-hip ratio are more useful indicators of central obesity. Values higher than the norms for your gender are more harmful to your heart health. The ideal waist circumference should not exceed 90 cm (35.5 in) for Asian males and 80 cm (31.5 in) in Asian females. For Caucasians, the cut-offs are 102 cm (40.2 in) for males and 88 cm (34.6 in) for females.

The waist-hip ratio is obtained by dividing the waist circumference by the hip circumference. The normal waist-to-hip ratio for Asians is less than 1.0 for men and less than 0.85 for women.

MANAGING OBESITY: METHODS OF LOSING WEIGHT
Diet and Exercise

Your body weight represents the balance between all the food calories you take in (energy input) and the calories you burn up in your daily activities (energy output). In order to lose weight and burn off fat, you need to get into a negative energy balance (less energy in than out). Basically, you will need to limit food intake and increase your activity level. Hard as it might seem initially, this mindset is the first step in a worthwhile pursuit.

You should then meet up with members of your diabetes care team, especially the dietitian, to work out a meal plan. A reduction in daily caloric intake by 500–1,000 kcal or limiting intake to 1,400–1,500 kcal daily is a reasonable start. You have to be absolutely honest with yourself. Consider cutting out your favourite snacks and eat low-fat foods.

The surest way to burn off the excess calories is doing regular aerobic exercises such as brisk walking, jogging, swimming, tennis, squash or badminton. Studies have shown that unless you enjoy the exercise, chances are you will soon give it up. Therefore, choose activities that you can sustain for a long time. If possible, exercise with a friend or partner who can motivate you. However there is the downside that such outings may turn out to be more social than calorie-burning. For more on exercise, see Chapter 3 Part 3.

Setting Goals for Exercise

Have a specific plan and set yourself realistic goals. Saying that you will exercise more is not specific enough. On the other hand, aiming to swim 20 laps every day is unrealistic for most people, unless you have your own swimming pool and a lot of stamina. Set more realistic goals, such as walking 30 minutes four times a week and gradually increasing this to 60 minutes every day.

Pacing Your Weight Reduction

In general, you should try to lose about 5% of your initial body weight by the end of three months, at a rate of 1–2 kg per month. For example, if you weigh 100 kg (220 pounds), a realistic target might be to try to reach 95 kg (210 pounds) in three months, and then go down to 90 kg (198 pounds) in another three months.

It is, of course, ideal to lose the targeted amount of weight. Do not, however, be discouraged if you seem to make less progress than you had planned to. Studies have shown that even if you do not reach your ideal weight for your height, any amount of weight loss is still valuable. In this situation, if your waist size has shrunk, that is a good sign. It indicates that you are burning excess fat but building a small amount of muscle and, hence, your weight has dropped only slightly. There is, most likely, a decrease in body fat and this will improve your blood sugar, cholesterol, triglycerides and blood pressure.

Maintaining Achieved Weight

It is very easy to regain the weight you have lost. When you have reached your target weight, try not to slacken but keep up the good work (and workouts). You may be tempted to reward yourself and catch up with some 'real' eating, but resist the temptation. Reward yourself, instead, with something non-fattening and inedible, such as a new dress or pair of pants (if your size has gone down, you are on the right track) or a DVD (but do not stay too long in front of the TV).

Medications

Weight-reduction medications are not 'quick fixes' for losing weight. Nonetheless, some of these prescription medications are approved for the overweight, especially those with other risk factors for heart disease and who have been shown to respond to diet and exercise but whose BMI is still hovering above 27 kg/m^2. For Asians, the cut-off BMI for starting anti-obesity drugs could be lowered to 25–27 kg/m^2.

Sibutramine or Reductil® acts on the brain to enhance satiety, making you less inclined to reach for that extra helping of dessert. Normally, when one loses weight, the body adapts by decreasing its metabolic rate. Sibutramine has the advantage that it dampens this adaptation, that is, it maintains your metabolic rate even as you start to lose weight. However, it may increase your blood pressure and, therefore, has to be used cautiously if you have hypertension.

Orlistat or Xenical® works by a different action. It reduces the absorption of fat in your food. Unabsorbed fat is passed out in the stool and this may sometimes be difficult to control, causing leakage of spots of oily faecal discharge. This can be minimised by increasing

Case 6: Mr ABM – Who Says You Cannot Lose Weight?

At age 20, Mr ABM weighed in at a hefty 154 kg and had a body mass index of 47 kg/m², having been obese since young. An infection of his genital area brought diabetes to his attention. Although he controlled his diabetes with oral medications, his weight languished between 154 to 161 kg, despite attempts at exercising and dieting. His doctors were prepared to put him through bariatric surgery (see below) to get his weight down to prevent complications of morbid obesity, but he backed out at the eleventh hour after he was informed of the potential side effects of the surgery.

He was spurred on to resume exercise and dieting. He would go to the Singapore Sports Complex to do treadmill running and to cycle and swim 2 to 3 hours a day. Within four months, he shed 22 kg (from 158 kg to 136 kg), and his HbA1c improved from 7.9% to 5.2% (whilst still taking metformin). Unfortunately, he could not keep up the pace and his weight gradually crept up to 156 kg. Undeterred, he resumed his efforts. He cut down on his carbohydrate and fat intake and ate more wholemeal bread, egg white, fish and fishballs, vegetables, fruits and lean chicken cuts. He would jog for 40 minutes and swim for an hour daily. Hitting 136 kg again, he was able to maintain it over the next eight months. When he last came for his checkup, his HbA1c was a nice 5.1%.

the consumption of fibre and continuing to keep to a low fat diet.

Used in conjunction with dietary measures, regular exercise and behavioural changes, these drugs have been proven effective and generally safe. But take them only under your doctor's supervision.

Surgery

Bariatric surgery may be recommended for morbidly obese individuals who fail to lose significant weight with diet, exercise and medications. For Asians, this means a BMI of at least 37.5 kg/m² (or 32.5 kg/m² if complications of obesity, such as diabetes, are already present). The corresponding BMI criteria for bariatric surgery for Caucasians are 40 kg/m² and 35 kg/m².

Bariatric operations are either to reduce stomach volume, thus giving earlier sensation of fullness and reducing food consumption, or creating a loop of gut for food to bypass the stomach and go straight to the intestines, or a combination of both. Their efficacy in weight reduction and improving diabetes control has been clinically proven. The improvement of diabetes with bariatric surgery goes beyond mere weight reduction; it preferentially alters several gut hormones and improves blood sugar levels. In 2010 bariatric surgery is considered an option, not just for treating obesity per se but also for treating diabetes. Bariatric surgery, however, is a last resort measure that is not without risk. It is undertaken only if the risk of the obesity and diabetes outweighs the risk of surgery. It is not an option for children and most adolescents, except in very extreme cases, and then only with parental consent.

COMMERCIAL SLIMMING PROGRAMMES?

The mass media carries many 'success' stories and glossy advertisements about new weight-loss treatments every day. They claim to produce weight-loss either by taking some pills or through a slimming programme.

Do be cautious, as many of these treatments are either anecdotal, ineffective over the long term, or are not scientifically proven. Many programmes that incorporate some kind of physical procedures, such as acupuncture and reflexology, actually combine quite drastic short-term calorie restriction. If effective, albeit in the short term, it will be due to the dietary component of the programme rather than the non-aerobic physical component. Advertisements highlight only the few successes and are silent about the many cases that did not work.

PART 2: EATING RIGHT

"Let your food be your medicine, and your medicine be your food".

—Hippocrates (460–375 BCE)
ancient Greek physician and the Father of Medicine

'Eating right' sounds good but the diabetic or overweight person soon realises that it is basically some form of diet control, which few people really like. But eating right is so important in the management of diabetes that we make no apologies for talking about it upfront.

Fundamental to the treatment of diabetes is an appropriate diet tailored to individual needs. This is regardless of whether you are taking diabetes tablets or insulin injections. A common mistaken concept is that dietary measures can be loosened up as long as medications are being taken.

You do not need special or expensive foods to control your diabetes. However, the wrong food choices or too much of certain foods may undo the effects of regular exercise and medications. Consistent self-discipline and will power is necessary for your long-term good. Your healthy food choices can also be a good influence on those around you!

The Role of Your Dietitian

Your dietitian will teach you the skills of eating right to achieve and maintain ideal body weight, blood sugar, blood lipids and blood pressure.

BALANCED REGULAR MEALS

Your diet should be appropriate in calorie content to achieve an ideal weight. It must be balanced, that is, it must have all the major food groups (carbohydrates, proteins, fats and micronutrients like minerals and vitamins) in the right quantity and quality.

In general, you will have to watch the amount of sugary foods, fats and salt you consume. Dietary fibres are generally encouraged. Protein restriction may be necessary if you have diabetic kidney disease.

Taking three well-spaced out meals is ideal. Snacks between the main meals are based on individual needs. This is to ensure that blood sugar levels do not fluctuate wildly. Irregular meals do not match the action profile of medications and can lead to times when blood sugar is too high or too low. For those who really cannot take well-spaced out meals, modifications to their medication schedule will have to be made on a case-by-case basis.

FOOD GROUPS: BASICS TO GO WITH YOUR MEALS
Let us start with the various food groups.

Carbohydrates
Carbohydrates are the primary and main source of sugar that gives you the energy to keep you alive and going. Every gram (g) of carbohydrate contains about 4 kilocalories (kcal). The amount of carbohydrates and calories you need depends on your state of diabetes, weight, age and activity level and special circumstances such as pregnancy and breastfeeding. The usual recommendation is to have 50–60% of total daily caloric intake in the form of carbohydrates.

Extremely low carbohydrate diets (less than 130 g per day) are not recommended in the management of diabetes, even when you are trying to lose weight. On the other hand, taking more carbohydrates than you need, relative to your energy output, will not only raise your blood sugar but make you put on weight. This is because unused carbohydrate is converted into glycogen and, eventually, fats which are stored in the liver, muscles and fat or adipose tissues.

Simple versus Complex Carbohydrates: the Difference
Both the amount and type of carbohydrates in food can influence blood sugar levels. Carbohydrates can be divided into simple carbohydrates (sugar) and complex carbohydrates (starch).

Simple carbohydrates or sugars are found in the form of glucose, syrup, honey, regular jams and sweets. Examples of complex carbohydrates are bread, rice, pasta, potato, fruits, milk and certain vegetables, such as carrots.

Simple carbohydrates are, in general, not suitable for people with diabetes as they are absorbed more quickly and cause a rapid rise in their blood sugar. They are to be eaten sparingly. The only time larger amounts of simple carbohydrates are acceptable is when one's blood sugar is low (hypoglycaemia) (see Chapter 6). Conversely, complex carbohydrates take longer to be digested and absorbed and, therefore, cause a more gradual and smaller rise in blood sugar, especially when taken with lots of dietary fibre. They give your pancreas more time to respond to the rising blood sugar.

Ways of Reducing Sugar Intake

Study the table below carefully. It lists the common food that contributes to your blood sugar. It is not uncommon that the first reaction to a question on how to reduce blood sugar is "I must cut down on meat and fried food". While meat and oily food should be taken in moderation (see the section on "Lipids" below), they do not, primarily, cause a rise in blood glucose. Instead, it is carbohydrate-rich food that raises your blood sugar.

1. Switching to low-sugar or sugar-free alternatives

Use Table 5 to help you reduce your carbohydrate consumption.

Table 5: Types of sugars to avoid and their better alternatives

Avoid	Better alternatives
White sugar, brown sugar, rock sugar, glucose, dextrose, sucrose, syrup, jam, honey, *kaya*, *gula melaka*, marmalade, condensed milk.	Artificial sweeteners e.g. Equal, Hermesetas, Sweetex, Pal Sweet, Lo-kal.
Sweets, chocolate, sweet biscuits, cakes, jelly, ice cream, *ice kachang*, *chendol*, canned fruits in syrup.	Plain crackers, wheat biscuits, desserts made with artificial sweetener, fresh fruits (in controlled portions).
Sugar-coated breakfast cereals, e.g. cocoa pops, honey-coated cereal.	High-fibre breakfast cereals e.g. oats, Weetabix, bran flakes, sugar-free muesli.
Ordinary fizzy drinks, soft drinks, sweetened fruit drinks, packet drinks, isotonic drinks, sweetened soy bean milk, flavoured milk drinks.	Diet soft drinks, Marmite, Bovril, clear soups, soda water, plain water, tea or coffee (with artificial sweetener).

Note: A description of the local food names (in italics) is available at the end of this chapter.

2. Using the carbohydrate exchange list

You don't have to live with a 'boring' diet. There is a wide range of foods that you can choose from. Refer to the carbohydrate exchange list (Table 6).

Each food and drink portion listed contains approximately 10 g of carbohydrate (also referred to as one carbohydrate portion). (Note, however, that some dietitians prefer to take one carbohydrate portion as 15 g.) The various portions may each be used to exchange one for the other in your meal plan to give you the same calories. The list is useful when you are looking at your meals in terms of portions. It allows you to estimate the consumed calories, since 1 g of carbohydrate gives you 4 kcal of energy. For example, one thin slice of bread can be substituted with two tablespoons of boiled rice, as both are 10 g of carbohydrate and give you about 40 calories (10 g × 4).

However, replacing one carbohydrate portion with another does not necessarily give you the same blood sugar rise after taking it. You are probably familiar with the experience that one portion of wholemeal bread gives you a smaller rise in blood glucose compared to one portion of white boiled rice. Therefore, when you make an exchange, it is advisable to test your blood glucose two hours after taking it. If it is too high, you may want to take a smaller portion of that carbohydrate, or try a different exchange.

Food experts attribute this to the difference in the glycaemic index (GI) of the various carbohydrates. The GI is a ranking of foods containing similar amounts of carbohydrate based on the rise in blood glucose after their consumption — the higher a food ranks in the GI, the higher the blood glucose rise. In general, go for those that rank low, or combine a low GI food with a high GI food to give an effect in the moderate GI range. If you want to know more about GI, speak to your dietitian.

Table 6: Carbohydrate exchange list

Cereals	One portion (10 g) is equivalent to
Bread (white or wholemeal)	1 thin slice
Rice (boiled)	2 tablespoons
Rice porridge	$^1/_2$ medium-size Chinese rice bowl
Noodles (cooked)	2 tablespoons
Beehoon (cooked)	2 tablespoons
Macaroni/spaghetti (cooked)	2 tablespoons

(continued on next page)

Instant oatmeal/rolled or raw oats (cooked)	2 tablespoons
Breakfast cereal e.g. bran flakes, corn flakes	3 tablespoons
Weetabix	1 biscuit
Chapati	¹/₂ size of teacup saucer
Thosai	¹/₃ size of dinner plate
Plain biscuits e.g. cream crackers or Marie biscuits	2 pieces
Plain (all-purpose) flour	1 level tablespoon
Corn flour	2 heaped teaspoons
Custard powder	2 heaped teaspoons
Fruits and Vegetables	**One portion (10 g) is equivalent to**
Apple, banana, orange, pear or starfruit	1 small fruit
Papaya, pineapple or melon	1 medium slice
Grapes	8–10
Jackfruit	2 seeds
Longans	8–10
Rambutans	3–4
Lychees	3–4
Watermelon	1 medium slice
Pomelo	2 sections
Baked beans (canned)	2 tablespoons
Red or green beans, lentils (cooked)	2 tablespoons
Potato, sweet potato	Size of an egg
Sweet corn	1 tablespoon
Yam (boiled)	2 level tablespoons
Milk and Milk Products	**One portion (10 g) is equivalent to**
Fresh milk (low-fat or skim)	1 glass (200 ml)
Milk powder (low-fat or skim)	5 heaped teaspoons
Yoghurt (low-fat and unsweetened)	1 small carton (200 g)
Evaporated (unsweetened)	¹/₂ glass (100 ml)
Fluid Exchange List	**One portion (10 g) is equivalent to**
Milk (fresh, pasteurised or low-fat)	1 glass (200 ml)
Malted or cocoa drinks (e.g. Horlicks, Milo, Ovaltine or cocoa)	2 heaped teaspoons
Orange juice (unsweetened)	¹/₂ glass (100 ml)
Rice porridge	¹/₂ medium Chinese bowl
Cream soup (canned or packet)	1 small teacup (200 ml)

Note: A description of the local food names (in italics) is available at the end of this chapter.

Oodles of good diabetes control[1]

Diabetrim® noodle (a scientifically engineered instant noodle for diabetics) contains fewer calories, less carbohydrates and fat, and more protein and fibre per 100 g compared to most ordinary 'non-diabetic' instant noodles. We conducted a controlled study at the Changi General Hospital on 30 Type 2 diabetic patients comparing Diabetrim® noodle with a well-established ordinary instant noodle brand. We found that the rise in blood glucose one hour after taking Diabetrim® noodle was 54% less than after taking the control noodle. After two hours, the rise in blood glucose was 59% less with Diabetrim® noodle (see graph below). The amount of carbohydrates and fibre in your meal therefore makes all the difference.

(Diabetrim® noodles can be obtained in Singapore in major pharmacies.)

Graph 1: Plasma glucose excursion after ingesting noodles

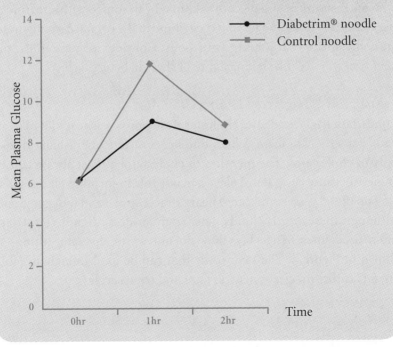

3. Using artificial sweeteners

Artificial sweeteners are allowed in your meal plan as they do not significantly raise your blood sugar.

There are two classes of artificial sweeteners. Nutritive or caloric sweeteners, as the name implies, have some calories. Taking too much of these, however, can add up to overall calorie intake and weight gain. Many snack items (cakes, chocolates, biscuits) labelled as 'suitable for diabetics' are sweetened with xylitol, sorbitol or fructose which contain about the same amount or half as much calories as glucose, weight for weight. Some of these sweeteners can also cause loose stools when taken in excess. In general, use these products in moderation.

The truly non-nutritive or non-caloric sweeteners, such as saccharin and aspartame, have only negligible calories and are, theoretically, better. Although there is no confirmed adverse health risk with these sweeteners, do stick to the acceptable daily intake (ADI), which is 5 mg per kg of body weight for saccharin and 40 mg per kg of body weight for aspartame.

Note that, although a piece of cake may be flavoured with an artificial sweetener, the flour and fat in it contribute to the overall carbohydrate, fat and calories that go into your body. Consider very carefully, the next time you feel like taking a bite of that 'diabetic cake'!

Lipids, Fats, Triglyceride and Cholesterol

Lipids, fats, triglyceride and cholesterol are words you hear a lot of from your diabetes care team. When one hears of fats one usually thinks only of cholesterol. The mention of cholesterol almost always causes anxiety because cholesterol plays a major role in forming plaques that clog up blood vessels and cause heart attack, stroke and foot gangrene. Although these words (lipids, fats, triglyceride and cholesterol) are often used interchangeably, they do not mean the same thing, as shown in Figure 4. The two words that can be used interchangeably are fats (more precisely, neutral fats) and triglyceride.

Figure 4: The composition of lipids

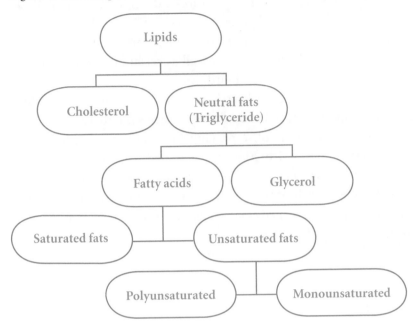

Lipids are a broad class of organic material in our body that includes fats and cholesterol. Cholesterol is chemically not a fat but a wax-like substance that is found in many types of food and also made in the liver. Dietary cholesterol contributes only about 15% of our body's cholesterol; the rest is made in the liver from fats. This is the reason why restricting cholesterol-rich food is sometimes not enough to keep your blood cholesterol in check and why medications are therefore needed. This is, however, no convenient excuse to let go of a controlled diet.

Fats refer to neutral fats or triglyceride, which is actually made up of a molecule of glycerol (itself derived from glucose) and three molecules of fatty acids.

That delicious piece of beefsteak that you might be eyeing certainly has lots of cholesterol, triglyceride and fatty acids.

Fatty acids can either be saturated fatty acids (or, simply, saturated fats) or unsaturated fatty acids (or, simply, unsaturated fats). Saturated fats are found abundantly in animal products (meat, butter, lard and ghee), as well as coconut and palm oil. They are solid at room temperature and when cold. Unsaturated fats, on the other hand, are liquid at room temperature and below. Unsaturated fats are either polyunsaturated or monounsaturated fats. They are found in relatively greater amounts in olive oil, canola oil, sunflower oil, peanut oil, corn oil, and soy oil as well as certain deep-sea fish, such as tuna, salmon, mackerel and sardines.

The metabolic link between triglyceride, fatty acids and cholesterol is very complex. Suffice to say that excessive saturated fats promote production of cholesterol, especially LDL-cholesterol (low-density lipoprotein cholesterol or the so-called 'bad' cholesterol). To make matters more complicated, there are many types of LDL-cholesterol particles. High levels of triglyceride promote the production of LDL-cholesterol particles called small-dense LDL-cholesterol that are more likely to clog up blood vessels.

Figure 5: The types of cholesterol

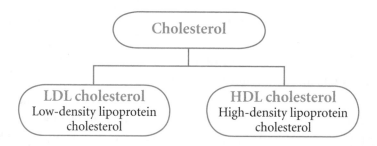

What about the so-called 'good' cholesterol or HDL-cholesterol (high-density-lipoprotein cholesterol)? The liver makes the protein envelope of these particles, which then circulate throughout the body to mop up the cholesterol from the tissues, including the blood vessels wall, forming HDL-cholesterol which is then taken up by the liver where it is metabolised and excreted into the bile.

Apart from saturated fat, trans fat is also bad for the heart, as it promotes the production of 'bad' cholesterol. Trans fat is produced when hydrogen is added to vegetable oil to increase the shelf life and stability of food and to enhance its taste. Trans fat can be found in vegetable shortenings, some margarines, crackers, cookies, snack foods, and other foods made with or fried in partially hydrogenated oils.

The Right Balance

For all their notoriety, fats and cholesterol are not all evil. You actually need them! Fat or adipose tissues serve as an insulator and a cushioning around organs. Fats and cholesterol are essential for the absorption of vitamins A, D, E and K, formation and maintenance of cell membranes, and production of bile and certain hormones.

Getting the right balance is the key. Fats are energy-rich. They pack in 9 kcal per gram compared to 4 kcal per gram of carbohydrate or protein. Therefore, unless you are able to burn away the calories, a high-fat diet will make it difficult for you to lose excess weight or maintain an ideal weight. Unused calories will be stored as triglyceride in the fat or adipose tissues. Note that cholesterol is itself not utilised for energy production.

1. General rules

Keep:
- Your weight in check
- Your LDL cholesterol down
- Your HDL cholesterol up
- Your triglyceride down

Eat:
- The right amount and type of fats
- Less cholesterol-rich food
- Less saturated fats (unsaturated fats are healthier)
- As little trans fat as possible

2. Recommendations

- Total daily fat intake should contribute only 20–30% of total daily calorie needs
- Saturated fat should be less than 10% of total fat intake
- Cholesterol intake should not exceed 300 mg per day

Tips on Reducing Fat and Cholesterol Intake

- Limit the intake of fried foods and choose clear soups instead of creamy ones.
- Use low-fat cooking methods, such as boiling, grilling, baking, roasting, stewing, steaming and microwave cooking.
- Use a non-stick frying pan to minimise the amount of oil needed for stir-frying.
- Trim off all visible fat and skin from meat and poultry.
- Limit the intake of full-cream dairy products as well as salad cream and mayonnaise.
- Use low-fat milk/skimmed milk instead of full-cream or coconut milk.
- Use low-fat cheese instead of full-cream / processed cheese.
- Remove saturated fat by refrigerating to solidify it and then removing the saturated fat.

Table 7: Better food choices

Limit	Better choice
Fried noodles/*bee hoon*/*mee*/*kway teow*	Noodles, *bee hoon, mee, kway teow* in soup or dry without oil and gravy. Avoid the fried onions and fried lard.
Fried rice, *briyani* rice, *nasi lemak*	Plain rice, unpolished rice and porridge with no added oil.
Roti prata, crisp *thosai*, *you tiao*, fried *popiah*	*Chapati, idli* with no ghee or oil, plain *popiah* with vegetable and lean meat filling
Laksa lemak, lontong	*Mee soto, soto ayam, yong tau foo* (non-fried pieces)
Curry dishes with heavy coconut milk	Curry dishes without coconut milk; use low-fat yoghurt or milk instead
Pig's trotter, roast pig with skin, poultry with skin	Lean meat, chicken/duck without skin
French fries	Boiled potato, baked/jacket potato
Salad with mayonnaise/ salad dressing	Fresh vegetable salad with vinegar, lime juice, or low-fat natural yoghurt

Note: A description of the local food names (in italics) is available at the end of this chapter.

Proteins

Proteins are essential nutrients used as building blocks to repair wear and tear of tissues and organs. They are also needed in the production of many hormones, enzymes and haemoglobin. Muscles and connective tissues are composed largely of proteins.

Proteins are made up of different amino acids linked together like strings of beads in varying sequence. Ingested proteins are broken down into their component amino acids which are then absorbed and distributed to all tissues to be linked up again to form different proteins. Because some of these amino acids cannot be made by the human body, they have to come from food sources and are therefore called essential amino acids. All the amino acids must be available at the same time for protein production.

Sources of Protein:

- Animal sources: milk, lean meat, poultry, egg white and fish. In general, they have all the amino acids, including the essential amino acids.
- Plant sources: beans, lentils, soy. Not all have essential amino acids; therefore vegetarians have to ensure that they eat not only the right amount but also from a variety of plant sources to prevent protein malnutrition.

The metabolism of proteins is closely integrated with those of carbohydrates and fats in very complex pathways. Proteins too provide calories. Like carbohydrate, each gram of protein gives about 4 kcal of energy. They can be converted in the liver into glucose when no glucose is coming in from the intestines, such as the period between dinner time and the next morning (assuming no post-dinner snacking). As proteins cannot be stored, excessive dietary protein is channelled into producing glucose and fats. This means excessive protein intake can also contribute to weight gain.

In a balanced diet, proteins typically make up 15–20% of the daily total calorie requirement.

Fibre

Dietary fibre is the non-digestible parts of foods. A high-fibre diet can improve your diabetic control because fibre slows down the rate of absorption of carbohydrates. It also makes you feel fuller and prevents overeating, and has the additional benefit of improving bowel function. You should attempt to take 20 g of fibre from a variety of food sources for every 1,000 kilocalories. (20-30 g of dietary fibre per day is the recommendation in the local context.)

Increasing Your Intake of Dietary Fibre

Choose high-fibre carbohydrate alternatives, as listed in Table 8.

Table 8: Low-fibre and high-fibre carbohydrates

Low-fibre carbohydrates	Higher fibre alternatives
White rice	Unpolished / brown rice
White bread	Wholemeal bread
Plain crackers	Wholewheat crackers
White pasta	Wholewheat pasta
White flour	Wholemeal flour
Corn flakes	Wheat biscuits (e.g. Weetabix), bran flakes, sugar-free muesli
Boiled potatoes	Boiled potatoes with skin, jacket potatoes
Pure fruit juice	Fresh fruit

Salt

High salt intake is associated with high blood pressure which increases the risk of stroke and heart disease. Take no more than 2 g of salt per day if you have high blood pressure. Everyone, diabetic or otherwise, will do well to keep salt intake to the minimum, unless he or she has a specific medical condition that requires more liberal salt consumption.

Tips to Reduce Salt Intake

- Use bottled sauces (such as oyster sauce, soy sauce, chilli and tomato sauce) sparingly.

- Avoid adding salt or sauces to cooked food or dipping food into sauces.
- Flavour food with spices and herbs (such as garlic, ginger, onions or lemon juice) instead of salt.
- Cut down on salty snacks (such as salted crisps and nuts).
- Minimise the consumption of canned meat, fish and soup.
- Choose fresh products rather than preserved products such as salted vegetables or salted meat/fish /eggs.

Vitamins and Minerals

Vitamins are essential micronutrients that have very varied functions. They help in the metabolism of carbohydrates, proteins and fats, acting, thus, as co-enzymes. Some vitamins, such as vitamin A, are essential for maintaining good eyesight, while others, like vitamin D, act more like a prohormone involved with calcium absorption.

Minerals such as sodium, potassium, chloride, calcium, phosphorus, magnesium, sulphur, etc. are essential components of the blood and tissues. Their roles are very varied—from maintaining fluid balance, bone and teeth strengthening, muscle contraction, nerve conduction to hormone production.

It is important that your 'diabetic' diet be balanced so that you have all these nutrients.

ALCOHOL

It is best to avoid alcohol altogether if you have diabetes. If you must drink, note that alcohol is relatively high in calories and should be used in moderation. Each gram of alcohol adds 7 kilocalories to your body, contributing to weight gain.

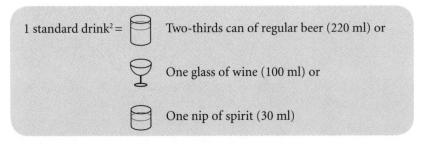

1 standard drink[2] = Two-thirds can of regular beer (220 ml) or

One glass of wine (100 ml) or

One nip of spirit (30 ml)

Dilute your drink with ice, diet drink or water to avoid over-consumption. Allow yourself no more than one drink per day, if you are an adult woman, or two per day, if you are a man. Each drink should contain not more than 15 g of alcohol.

Alcohol should not be taken on an empty stomach. This is because when a proper meal is not taken and the diabetic person develops hypoglycaemia, alcohol in the body makes it harder for the liver to make and release glucose to counter the hypoglycaemia, thus prolonging it. Furthermore, the effects of alcohol, such as speech incoherence or drowsiness, are hard to differentiate from those of hypoglycaemia.

If your triglyceride is high, alcohol will raise it even further and this may cause pancreatitis or inflammation of the pancreas. Repeated attacks of pancreatitis will lead to further reduction of insulin reserves and worsen diabetes. If you have diabetic neuropathy (see Chapter 2), alcohol will worsen it.

Case 7: Mr IT – Surviving Four Festive Seasons

Mr IT resisted an increase in the dose of his oral diabetes medications when his HbA1c was in the range of 7.9 to 8.1%, promising to be stricter on his diet. Stricter he was, from October 07 to February 08. In his own words, through 'four festive seasons' (Deepavali, Hari Raya Puasa, Christmas and Chinese New Year), he resisted all the festive goodies and ate less rice at dinner. His HbA1c improved to 7.1%. This shows that a lot can be achieved if you watch your diet!

THE HEALTHY DIET PYRAMID

The Healthy Diet Pyramid is for everybody, not just people with diabetes. It is not difficult to commit it to memory.

Figure 6: The Healthy Diet Pyramid

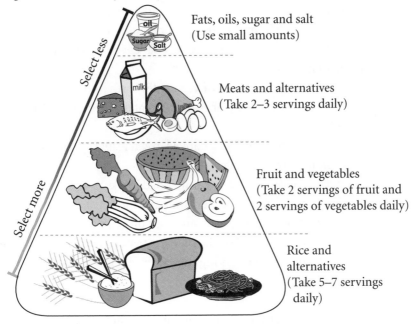

To eat healthily, most of the food should come from the base and the least from the tip of the Healthy Diet Pyramid.

There are basically four food groups, namely:

a. Rice and alternatives
b. Fruit and vegetables
c. Meat and alternatives
d. Fats, oils, sugar and salt

Choose a variety of food from each food group and only use food items from the top of the pyramid sparingly for flavouring.

For the diabetic person, the general guidelines are as follows:

- Rice and alternatives. This should make up the main component of the diet and the amount depends on the carbohydrate portions recommended by your dietitian. Use the carbohydrate exchange list as a guide if you need to.

- Fruits. Fruits are great sources of vitamins, minerals, dietary fibre and phytochemicals. The recommended intake is two servings of fruits per day and, again, you may use the carbohydrate exchange list to help you with what type of fruits to select and the amount to eat.
- Vegetables. These are very important and valuable sources of beta-carotene, vitamin C, dietary fibre and other phytochemicals. Dark green leafy vegetables are good sources of iron, folate and calcium.
  A minimum of two servings of vegetables is recommended, although more of the leafy ones may be eaten if required. One serving (or
  ¾ mug) is equivalent to 150 g cooked green leafy vegetables or 100 g of non-leafy vegetables.
- Meat and alternatives. The recommended intake is 2–3 servings per day. These food items such as meat, fish, poultry, bean curd and beans are great sources of protein.
- Fats, oils, sugar and salt. For the diabetic person, sugar should be avoided while food items high in fats and oils should only be used sparingly for flavouring.

In summary, a diabetic diet is a healthy diet. Based on your carbohydrate/diet allowance, use the Healthy Diet Pyramid as a guide to help you select your food to enjoy a variety of food items and still stay healthy!

TRY IT OUT—GO AHEAD AND EXPERIMENT

Frankly, it is not always easy to know how much or what to eat to keep your weight, sugar and lipid levels in healthy balance. This chapter would, however, have served its purpose if you are now more conscious of what you eat, have a better understanding of what your doctor, nurse and dietitian are trying to convey to you, and start to look at food labels.

The surest way is to try out a particular food portion and check your blood sugar about two hours later to see if it falls within the acceptable range (see Chapter 5). If it consistently gives you high readings, what you have to do next is to reduce the portion or make a switch to something else. What you must *not* do is tell yourself, "I know four seeds of durian will surely shoot my glucose through the roof, therefore I will not test."

Description of local food

bee hoon	rice vermicelli
chapati	grilled Indian flat bread made with atta (100%) whole wheat flour
chendol	a dessert of green pea flour strips, red beans and coconut cream
gula melaka	palm sugar
ice kachang	a shaved ice, sweetened dessert
idli	a savoury pancake of steamed batter consisting of dehusked black lentils and rice
kaya	coconut egg jam
kway tiao	flat rice noodles
laksa lemak	noodles in rich coconut gravy
lontong	rice cakes in coconut milk gravy
mee	yellow noodles
mee rebus	yellow noodles in sweet potato gravy, with tofu and egg
mee soto	spicy chicken noodle soup
nasi lemak	coconut-flavoured rice
popiah	spring roll stuffed with turnip strips, prawn and eggs
roti prata	thick, flat Indian bread made with wheat flour, sugar, salt and water and fried in oil or ghee
soto ayam	spicy chicken soup with rice cubes
thosai	thin pancake made with fermented rice and gram batter
yong tau foo	tofu and vegetables stuffed with fish paste
you tiao	crullers or fried dough fritters

PART 3: EXERCISE

*"I am always doing that which I cannot do
in order that I may learn how to do it."*

—*Pablo R. Picasso (1881–1973)*
Spanish artist, painter and sculptor

The mention of physical exercise often sparks off reactions like "no time", "too tired by the time I finish work", "too troublesome", "it's been raining/too hazy". It is, therefore, useful to remind ourselves of the following general benefits of exercise:
- Promotes weight loss in the overweight
- Lowers the risk of heart attack by reducing body fats and blood pressure
- Increases muscle strength and flexibility
- Improves physical endurance
- Relieves stress
- Enhances a sense of well-being

For people with pre-diabetes and diabetes, exercise holds a special role in management because exercise:
- Reduces insulin resistance
- Prevents diabetes
- Lowers blood glucose and improves diabetes control
- Reduces insulin or oral medication requirements
- Lowers triglyceride and raises HDL-cholesterol ('good' cholesterol)

INCIDENTAL EXERCISE
You do not need special preparations for incidental exercise. You only need the right mindset. As far as time permits, build as much incidental physical activities into your daily routine as possible. Take the stairs instead of the lift, walk or cycle to the neighbourhood shop instead of taking the car, park further away from the entrance to the supermarket.

STARTING AN EXERCISE PROGRAMME

In addition to incidental exercise, embark on a regular exercise programme. This does require some planning and personal sacrifice but it is well worth the effort. There are, however, some constraints and precautions that you should observe if you have diabetes.

A full assessment of your diabetes is recommended to determine your current diabetes control and whether you have any diabetic complications which may not allow you to do certain activities. You may need to undergo specific tests for heart disease, depending on your doctor's judgement of your current risk.

Exercise should be started cautiously. Gradually increase the intensity and duration as you get fitter. The desired intensity varies, depending on whether your goal is to lose weight, increase strength, improve muscle and joint flexibility and mobility, or improve physical fitness. It is also determined by individual preference and limitations.

Types of Exercise

Aerobic activities are those that move major muscle groups, can be sustained for minutes to hours, and increases your heart rate. Examples include walking, cycling, jogging, swimming, dancing and tennis.

Resistance exercises are brief and intense and cannot be sustained for more than a few seconds or minutes, such as weight training. They increase strength, muscle bulk and metabolic rate.

Both types of exercise will reduce insulin resistance and complement each other to lower your blood sugar. If you exercise regularly and your diabetes is already well-controlled, you might be able to lower your medication dosage and still remain in good control. If it is not well controlled, the exercise might just give you that extra something that you need to improve it.

Exercise Frequency and Intensity

The recommendation is 150 minutes of moderate aerobic physical activity per week. This intensity level means working your heart rate to 50–70% of the maximum for one's age (see the calculations below). Space out the exercise. Exercise for at least 30 minutes on most or all days of the week, taking no more than two consecutive days of break.

A minimum of five times a week is recommended for weight loss and three times a week for weight maintenance and improving fitness. The recommendation for resistance exercise, if not contraindicated, is three times a week.

If you are exercising to lose weight, start with aerobic exercises and introduce resistance exercises when you are nearing or have achieved your weight-loss target.

If your fitness level is very low, start with a shorter duration of 10–15 minutes. This can be gradually increased to three 10–15-minute sessions spread out over the day, although this may not be practical for most people.

Two simple ways to gauge your exercise intensity:
1. Talk test. If you cannot whistle or talk during the activity, you are exercising too hard. If you can either whistle or talk continuously, the activity is not intensive enough to achieve target heart rate. Aim for something in between.
2. Heart rate. Aim for a heart rate of 50–70% of your estimated maximum heart rate, which is 220 minus your age. For example, if you are 45 years old, your maximum heart rate is $220 - 45 = 175$. 60% of maximum heart rate is $(60 \times 175) / 100 = 105$ beats/minute.

(Note: Take note that this calculation does not take into account your specific health condition or medications that can alter the response of heart rate to exercise.)

To avoid injury, aerobic exercise should always be preceded by 5–15 minutes of static stretching and low intensity aerobics of the muscles that you are working during the actual activity. At the end of the exercise you should slow down the pace for 10 minutes to cool down.

Timing of Exercise

The only reason why exercising in the morning is usually recommended is that the air is still fresh at that time of the day. Apart from this, exercising 90 to 120 minutes after a meal is more logical, as it is the time when your blood sugar normally peaks. You can use the exercise to bring down your blood sugar. This is not always practical, however, so exercise when it is convenient.

EXERCISE AND BLOOD GLUCOSE MONITORING

It is always a good habit to check your blood glucose before, during (if the exercise is strenuous and prolonged), and after the activity, unless you are doing the same routine that has proven previously not to have caused any disruption to your blood sugar. Therefore, if you change the exercise type and intensity, or have recently changed your oral diabetes medication or insulin, or even insulin injection site, start all over again and check your blood sugar as recommended.

If at any time during your exercise, you experience symptoms of hypoglycaemia, stop and check your blood sugar level. As the effects of moderate exercise on your blood sugar can extend beyond the first few hours after the activity, look out for hypoglycaemia and test your blood sugar when necessary. It is better to over-test than under-test. All this might seem like a chore, but once you have settled into a routine, it not only becomes easier, but you will be happier for the good it does to your sugar level.

Safety Rules

- For Type 1 diabetes, if your blood sugar is over 14 mmol/L, check your urine for ketones. You may proceed with the exercise if you feel well and the urine ketone test is negative. If, however, the test is positive, your body is not having enough insulin. You will then need additional insulin to bring down your sugar level. Do not exercise until the ketone test becomes negative. Exercising when the blood glucose is high and ketones are present in the urine can raise the blood sugar even higher owing to the release of stress hormones during the activity.
- On the other hand, as a general rule, if your blood sugar level is below 5.6 mmol/L, take a 15 g carbohydrate snack. Test again 15 minutes later. Do not start exercising until your blood sugar level is above 5.6 mmol/L.

EXERCISE AND DIABETES MEDICATIONS
Insulin Injections

Exercising when one is on insulin can be tricky business but should not deter you from doing so. Here are some general points to note to enjoy your exercise.

- Choose injection sites that are less likely to be affected by the working muscles. Insulin is absorbed faster at the exercising part of the body. For example, if insulin has been given in the thigh, walking, jogging or cycling can cause faster and greater absorption of insulin and this may lead to hypoglycaemia.
- Exercise during peak insulin action is also more likely to cause hypoglycaemia. If exercising during the peak of insulin action is anticipated or planned, the appropriate insulin dose can be reduced. If it is unplanned, extra carbohydrates should be taken before the activity.
- Keep records of your insulin and snack adjustments, so that you can use them to analyse the effects of the exercise on your blood glucose.

Some exercise safety tips
- Check your blood sugar before, during and after exercise
- Have immediate access to simple carbohydrates (such as glucose tablets) to treat hypoglycaemia during and after exercise
- Drink sufficient fluids to prevent dehydration
- Exercise with a friend who knows how to recognise and treat hypoglycaemia
- Wear or carry with you some form of diabetes identification
- Stop exercising if you experience:
  Light-headedness or dizziness
  Chest tightness / heaviness / discomfort / pain
  Severe shortness of breath
  Nausea

Oral Medications

Hypoglycaemia is less of a problem if you are taking only oral medications, but may still occur if you are taking any that acts by stimulating release of insulin, such as sulphonlyurea or metiglinide. The dose may then have to be reduced, especially if you are exercising at the peak action of the drug. The case at the end of this chapter illustrates this point. If you are not taking either of these types of diabetes drugs, hypoglycaemia is unlikely to occur with exercise.

If you have hypoglycaemia that you suspect is related to exercise, discuss it with your doctor.

EXERCISE AND PRE-EXISTING DIABETES COMPLICATIONS

Heart Disease

If you have pre-existing heart disease, a heart check by a cardiologist is recommended to determine your fitness and whether you should start with a graduated exercise under medical supervision.

Retinopathy

If you have severe diabetic eye disease (diabetic retinopathy), avoid vigorous aerobic or resistance exercise as it may trigger vitreous haemorrhage or retinal detachment. Swimming and cycling are preferred to spot running. Avoid exercise that positions your eyes below your heart level, e.g. touching your toes.

Peripheral Neuropathy

Decreased pain sensation in the feet increases the risk of injury. Avoid full- weight bearing exercises, such as running and skipping. Swimming, cycling or arm exercises are safer. Always wear well-fitting shoes and check your feet after the exercise for redness, cuts or open sores.

Autonomic Neuropathy

Diabetics with autonomic neuropathy should undergo a health check before starting more vigorous unaccustomed exercise. This is because it can cause silent heart attack, poor heart and respiratory response to exercise and poor body temperature regulation.

Diabetic Kidney Disease

Diabetic kidney disease occurs in stages, starting with the appearance of small amounts of protein in the urine. Physical activity can increase the amount of protein in the urine but this, by itself, is of no consequence. There is, however, no evidence that vigorous exercise increases the rate of progression of diabetic kidney disease and hastens kidney failure. There is no specific exercise restriction for people with diabetic kidney disease, unless he or she is already suffering from kidney failure. You may do mild exercises, such as walking, if you do not have advanced kidney failure.

Case 8: Mr LFK – Exercising Safely

Mr LFK, a 50-year-old Type 2 diabetic, had stenting of his coronary blood vessels done for a heart attack six months ago. He underwent uneventful, supervised cardiac rehabilitation exercise at the hospital and lost 6 kg of his original weight of 78 kg and felt generally fitter after three months. He then began 45–60 minutes of brisk walking four times a week on his own.

However, he was beginning to experience mild light-headedness during the exercise and after. Fortunately, he had been checking his blood glucose regularly. His doctor noticed that four recent readings were below 3.5 mmol/L, either during or 1–2 hours after the exercise. Readings at other times were within a nice range of 4.5–7 mmol/L.

He treated his hypoglycaemia with orange juice followed by a chocolate wafer bar, as his next meal was not until two hours later. Mr LFK saw his weight creeping up again. His doctor replaced one of his two types of diabetes pills with one that was less likely to cause low blood glucose and Mr LFK was, thus, able to continue his exercise routine without hypoglycaemia.

Comments:
1. Exercise is beneficial for cardiac fitness, weight control and glucose control.
2. Hypoglycaemia can occur with exercise, especially after you have successfully attained cardiac fitness.
3. Hypoglycaemia can be harmful to your heart, especially if you have already had a heart attack.

4. Frequent hypoglycaemia and treatment with excessive carbohydrates can result in weight gain.
5. Checking blood glucose before and after exercise is important. The effect of exercise can last for more than 24 hours. Hence, look out for hypoglycaemia beyond the immediate few hours after exercise.
6. Taking a carbohydrate snack before, during and after exercise helps to avoid hypoglycaemia but may make you put on weight.
7. A review and change of your diabetes medication may be necessary to avoid exercise-induced hypoglycaemia. In the above case, the switch was from taking glibenclamide twice a day to taking glimepiride once a day (see Chapter 3 Part 4).
8. Once you have maintained a pattern, you may do less blood glucose checks, but any unaccustomed exercise or increase in intensity requires more precautionary checks.

Case 9: Mr SG – Hypoglycaemia due to Increased Physical Activity

Mr SG, 53 years old, had diabetes for four years and was taking gliblenclamide (5 mg in the morning and 2.5 mg at dinner time) and metformin (250 mg twice daily) and was doing fairly well with a HbA1c of 7.6%. His exercise routine was usually 30 to 45 minutes of brisk walking prior to dinner. One day, he decided to exercise after dinner and for 90 minutes. That night, he developed 'hypo' in the middle of the night with palpitations and cold sweat. The symptoms were relieved by taking bread and Milo.

Comments: An increase in the level of physical activity can certainly lead to 'hypo'. To prevent it you should take extra carbohydrates after the activity and ensure that at bedtime, your blood glucose is at least 5 mmol/L.

Figure 7: The Activity Pyramid details physical activities that can be done regularly as part of a healthy lifestyle.

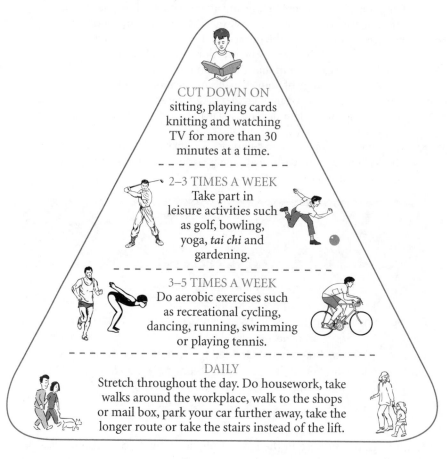

CUT DOWN ON
sitting, playing cards knitting and watching TV for more than 30 minutes at a time.

2–3 TIMES A WEEK
Take part in leisure activities such as golf, bowling, yoga, *tai chi* and gardening.

3–5 TIMES A WEEK
Do aerobic exercises such as recreational cycling, dancing, running, swimming or playing tennis.

DAILY
Stretch throughout the day. Do housework, take walks around the workplace, walk to the shops or mail box, park your car further away, take the longer route or take the stairs instead of the lift.

PART 4: ORAL DIABETES MEDICATIONS

"Let your food be your medicine, and your medicine be your food."

—Hippocrates (460–375 BCE)
ancient Greek physician and the Father of Medicine

Oral diabetes medications are mainly used for the treatment of Type 2 diabetes. They are prescribed when dietary measures and physical exercise fail to bring the blood sugar to the desired level. It is important to understand that oral medications are to supplement and not to totally replace prudent eating and regular exercise.

The different diabetes pills work in different ways and have different side effects. They may be used singly or in combination to give you the desired results. The dose and dosing schedule depend on the medication and your specific needs.

Figure 8 shows the main sites of action of commonly used oral diabetes drugs. They stimulate insulin secretion, reduce liver glucose production, promote glucose uptake by muscles and fat cells or reduce intestinal absorption of carbohydrates.

Figure 8: The main sites of action of commonly used oral diabetes drugs

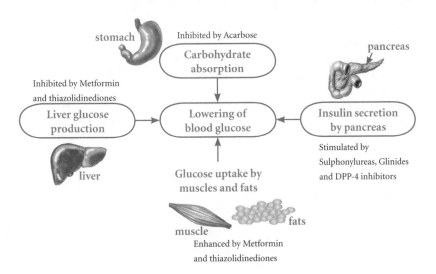

Check the medications you are taking against Table 9 to better understand how they work.

Your doctor will make an initial assessment of your diabetes based on many factors: duration of diabetes, your blood sugar trend and current level, your weight, whether you have symptoms, and any other concurrent illnesses, just to name a few. He may, then, decide to treat your diabetes just with dieting and regular exercise. On the other hand, if your blood sugar is very high, you will need insulin, even if you are a Type 2 diabetic and have only just been diagnosed. He may later stop the insulin and switch to tablets. Any state in between these two extremes would be treated with one or two types of tablets, initially. The dose will then be adjusted depending on your body's response to and tolerance of the pills. If the desired blood sugar target is not reached, your doctor may prescribe up to three (rarely four) types of pills at maximum doses.

Taking diabetes pills is no licence to slacken on your diet and regular exercise. The good news is that if you are overweight, shedding some of that fat through lifestyle changes may allow your doctor to reduce the dose of diabetes medications.

Table 9: Diabetes medications

Medications	How they work	Timing and frequency	Additional information and side effects
Drug Class			
Insulin secretagogues (a) Sulphonylureas Glibenclamide Gliclazide Glimepiride Glipizide Tolbutamide	Stimulate pancreas to release insulin.	Immediately before to 30 minutes before meals. Tolbutamide: twice or thrice daily; The rest—once or twice daily.	Tends to cause weight gain. Alcohol interferes with these tablets and may result in side effects, such as vomiting and flushing of the face.

(b) Meglitinides Nateglinide Repaglinide	Stimulate pancreas to release insulin.	Immediately before each main meal. Thrice daily with each main meal.	Meglitinides have a rapid onset of action and short duration of action. If you skip a meal, skip the dose for that meal.
Biguanides Metformin	Reduces the liver's production of glucose and increases the uptake of glucose by muscles and fat tissues.	Immediately after meals. Once to thrice daily depending on individual needs.	May cause gastrointestinal side effects like abdominal pain and diarrhoea. These side effects are dose-dependent and tend to go away with time. Metformin may cause some weight loss and may reduce the absorption of vitamin B_{12}.
Alpha-glucosidase inhibitors Acarbose	Delays the digestion and absorption of carbohydrates and slows the rise of blood glucose after a meal.	With the first mouthful or immediately before each main meal. Once to thrice a day depending on individual needs. Usually taken with each main meal.	Diarrhoea, abdominal discomfort and flatulence (gas) are common side effects. These are usually mild and can be minimised by gradual dosing, and may go away with time.
Thiazolidinediones Rosiglitazone Pioglitazone	Improve insulin sensitivity (i.e. reduce insulin resistance) in muscles and fat tissues and reduce the liver's production of glucose.	Timing in relation to meals is not crucial but it is advisable to take this class of medication at the same time each day. Once or twice daily.	May cause weight gain, anaemia and leg oedema (swelling due to water retention). May worsen pre-existing heart failure and increase the risk of cardiac ischaemia[*,1,2].

DPP-4 Inhibitors Sitagliptin Vildagliptin	Stimulate insulin and suppress glucagon secretion by enhancing the effects of a group of gut hormones called incretins.	Timing in relation to meals is not crucial but it is advisable to take this class of medication at the same time each day. Once or twice daily.	This is the latest class of anti-diabetes drugs. They do not cause weight gain.
Combination medications Rosiglitazone with metformin Glibenclamide with metformin Sitagliptin and metformin Vildagliptin and metformin	Taken once or twice daily depending on individual needs. Actions and side effects are similar to those of the individual component medications (glibenclamide, rosiglitazone, metformin, sitagliptin, vildagliptin). They cut down the number of pills that need to be taken, but, as the dose of the individual component drugs is fixed, dose adjustment is less flexible.		

*This precaution arose from a report in the *New England Journal of Medicine* in May 2007.[1] The report, based on a meta-analysis of 42 trials, suggested an increase in heart attacks in patients who took rosiglitazone, although there were arguably some inherent weakness in the study. A subsequent analysis of three large randomized controlled prospective trials was not conclusive on the matter. While the initial report did not, therefore, lead to a withdrawal of the drug from the market, the manufacturer has been asked by the US Food and Drug Administration (or FDA) to conduct a long-term study to further evaluate the safety of this drug.

It also resulted in various health regulatory authorities mandating that the drug package insert includes information on the potential risk of cardiac ischaemia with its use.[2]

At the time of this reprint, there has been no new data on the subject.

Some General Guidelines when Taking Your Oral Diabetes Medication

- Know the name and dosage of your diabetes medicine.
- Take your medications at the correct time and at the correct doses. Do not make any changes to your medication routine without consulting your diabetes care team.
- Do not miss or delay meals, otherwise your blood sugar may drop too low.

- Take your diabetes medication(s) even when you are sick. (Sometimes the dose may have to be adjusted.)
- Other medications can interact with diabetes tablets. Check with your doctor or pharmacist before taking other medications, including over-the-counter ones.
- If you forget to take a dose, take the missed dose as soon as you remember. However, if it is almost time for the next dose, skip the missed dose and continue with your regular dosing schedule. Do not take a double dose to make up for a missed dose.
- Inform your doctor if you experience or notice any of the following symptoms (as they may indicate adverse effects): loss of appetite, yellowing of eyes or skin (jaundice), dark or tea-coloured urine, light-coloured stools, diarrhoea, nausea or vomiting, unexplained fever and sore throat, itching or skin rash, increased sensitivity to sunlight, and frequent hypoglycaemia (see Chapter 6)

Limitations of Oral Diabetes Medications

- If you are undergoing surgery or have an acute illness such as infection or injury, insulin may be needed to temporarily bring down very high sugar levels to help you combat the infection and prepare you for surgery.
- Pregnant women with Type 2 diabetes who are on oral diabetes drugs will have to switch to insulin during pregnancy, as diabetes pills are currently not recommended in pregnancy.
- Finally, Type 2 diabetes is, unfortunately, a progressive disease, that is, with time the insulin reserve in the pancreas declines further to a stage where oral diabetes drugs are no longer able to maintain normal blood sugar. Insulin will then be permanently needed (see Chapter 3 Part 5).

PART 5: INSULIN THERAPY AND INCRETIN ANALOGUES

*"The man who can drive himself further
once the efforts get painful is the man who will win."*

*—Sir Roger G. Bannister (1929–)
English athlete, first to run the mile in under four minutes*

Insulin is a hormone produced by the beta-cells of the islets of Langerhans in the pancreas. One of its main functions is the regulation and maintenance of normal blood glucose.

WHO NEEDS INSULIN?

1. Type 1 diabetics
2. Type 2 diabetics under the following situations:
   - When blood sugar can no longer be adequately controlled with diet, exercise and oral medications because the pancreas is no longer producing enough insulin.
   - During Diabetic Ketoacidosis (DKA) or Hyperosmolar Hyperglycaemia Syndrome (HHS).
   - During an intercurrent event that makes the diabetes temporarily go out of control, such as injury, infection, heart attack or major surgery.
   - In preparation for pregnancy (pre-conception) and during pregnancy (see Chapter 14 for more details on this subject).

TYPES OF INSULIN

Current insulin therapy is by injection. Oral insulin is a dream of all diabetics who need insulin but its successful development is still a distant prospect. Insulin inhaled into the lungs is still finding its footing (see page 80). Meanwhile, diabetics who need insulin will have to put up with injections.

Case 10: Mr TYM – Going on Insulin to Feel Better

Mr TYM is 76 years old and has had Type 2 diabetes for 30 years with complications. He had a heart attack for which he had coronary bypass surgery and poor blood circulation and neuropathy in his feet, causing numbness. His diabetes was in poor control (HbA1c 11.5% and a random non-fasting blood glucose of 21 mmol/L, despite taking two types of diabetes oral medications). He had increased urination, excessive thirst and had lost 5 kg in just over two weeks. He was thus started on insulin.

Within two months, he had regained 4 kg and felt better. He had more stamina, was sleeping and eating better, and was doing treadmill walking exercises daily. He no longer had to get up in the middle of the night to empty his bladder. His urine sugar tests (which used to show a brown reaction indicating lots of sugar) were now giving a blue reaction indicating no sugar in the urine. His HbA1c was now below 8.0% on a total of 40 units of insulin given in two daily injections. Although there is still a role for urine sugar tests, as they are cheaper, Mr TYM agreed to switch to testing blood sugar instead, because urine sugar indicates when your blood sugar is high but not when it is low and, therefore, cannot warn him of hypoglycaemia.

There are several types of insulin available. Insulin used to be derived from pigs (porcine insulin) or cows (beef insulin) and these are still used in some countries. Nowadays, most parts of the world, including Singapore, use genetically engineered human insulin, which is structurally similar to our own body's insulin.

Besides human insulin, there are also many different insulin analogues, which are human insulin molecules that have been chemically modified, resulting in changed physical, chemical and physiological properties. Examples of insulin analogues are insulin lispro (Humalog®), insulin aspart (NovoRapid®), insulin glulisine (Apidra®), insulin glargine (Lantus®) and insulin detemir (Levemir®).

The various types of insulin and insulin analogues differ in how quickly they start to work (onset of action), the time taken to reach their maximum or peak action and how long they continue to lower blood glucose (duration of action).

In someone without diabetes, insulin switches on and off according to the prevailing blood sugar. When the blood sugar is high (after a meal, for example), it switches on, but in a state of fast it switches off, thus maintaining the blood glucose in a narrow physiological range.

Although the objective of insulin therapy is to normalise blood glucose, keeping blood sugar within the normal physiological range at all times is difficult, if not impossible. This is because once injected, the insulin cannot be switched off anytime we want it to. An insulin regimen (type of insulin, dose, frequency and time of injection) is, therefore, chosen to fit individual needs. In general, this regimen should be able to deal with the rise in blood sugar after a meal and to provide enough basal insulin to keep the blood sugar normal or acceptable throughout the day.

In order to individualise treatment, your doctor will choose from a wide range of insulins available. The table below shows the properties of the various insulins. Study it to understand the action profile of the insulin(s) you are currently using.

Table 10: Injectable insulins and insulin analogues

Insulin	Brands	Onset of action	Time to peak action	Duration of action
Regular (short-acting)	Food must be taken within 30 to 45 minutes of injection			
Soluble insulin	Actrapid HM®	30 min	1–3 hr	6–8 hr
	Humulin R®	30 min	2–4 hr	6–8 hr
Rapid-acting	Insulin Aspart and Insulin Lispro: Food must be taken within 10 minutes of injection in order to prevent low blood sugar (hypoglycaemia). Insulin glulisine (Apidra®): Can be injected up 15 minutes before or 20 minutes after a meal.			
Insulin Aspart	NovoRapid®	10–20 min	1–3 hr	3–5 hr
Insulin Lispro	Humalog®	5–15 min	½–1½ hr	3–5 hr
Insulin Glulisine	Apidra®	10–15 min	½–1 hr	2–4 hr

(continued on next page)

Intermediate-acting	Food must be taken within 30 to 45 minutes of injection			
Isophane Insulin (NPH)	Humulin N®	1–2 hr	6–12 hr	18–24 hr
	Insulatard HM®	1½ hr	4–12 hr	18–24 hr
Lente or Insulin Zinc Suspension (IZS)	Humulin L®	1–3 hr	6–12 hr	18–24 hr
Long-acting	Time of injection in relation to food or meal is not crucial, but should be given around the same time each day.			
Extended Insulin Zinc Suspension (IZS)	Humulin U®	3 hr	6–14 hr	up to 24 hr
	Ultratard®	4 hr	8–24 hr	22–28 hr
Insulin Glargine	Lantus®	2 hr	Peakless	continuous basal action
Insulin Detemir	Levemir®	1 hr	6–8 hr	up to 24 hr
Combination	Timing of meals after injection is dependent on whether regular short-acting or rapid-acting insulin is used in the combination mixture			
Mixture of 25% Insulin Lispro (rapid-acting) and 75% protaminated Insulin Lispro (intermediate acting)	Humalog Mix 25®	5–15 min	Dual phase Early peak occurs after ½-1 hour	up to 22 hr
Mixture of 30% Insulin Aspart (rapid-acting) and 70% protaminated Insulin Aspart (intermediate-acting)	NovoMix 30®	10–20 min	1–4 hr	up to 24 hr
Mixture of 30% Regular (short-acting) Insulin and 70% Isophane Insulin (intermediate-acting)	Humulin 30/70®	30 min	1–5 hr	10–24 hr
	Mixtard 30 HM®	30 min	2–8 hr	up to 24 hr
Mixture of 50% Regular (short-acting) Insulin and 50% Isophane Insulin (intermediate-acting)	Mixtard 50 HM®	30 min	2–8 hr	up to 24 hr

*Isophane insulin is synonymous with NPH (Neutral Protamine Hagedorn). It contains zinc and protamine.

(continued on next page)

Notes:
1. This table serves only as a reference. Information is based on subcutaneous injection. Insulin effects vary from patient to patient.
2. Low blood sugar (hypoglycaemia) is more likely to occur around the time of maximum or peak action. Blood sugar may remain high (hyperglycaemia) before the insulin starts acting, or when its action is ending.
3. The combination insulins are pre-mixed solutions of either regular short-acting or rapid-acting insulin plus intermediate-acting insulin. Using these combination insulins avoids the need to mix the two forms of insulin in the syringe. The disadvantage is that they have a fixed ratio of the two component insulins and, therefore, may not be suitable for all patients.

Graph 2: Insulin action times

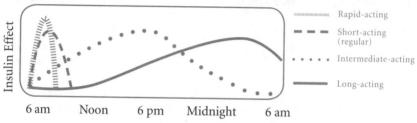

INSULIN DELIVERY DEVICES

There are several devices that can be used to deliver insulin. A few of these are briefly described here.

Syringes

Insulin is commonly injected using a syringe with a needle attached. Syringes are used to accurately draw out the insulin from the insulin container or vial. Choose a suitable syringe that allows you to draw out the amount you are using. Insulin is measured in units. A 0.3 mL syringe allows you to draw out 30 units maximum, a 0.5 mL syringe, 50 units and a 1 mL syringe, 100 units. This information is stated on the packaging. Although you can use a higher volume syringe (e.g. 0.5 ml syringe) to draw out a small amount of insulin (e.g. 10 units) it will be more accurate if you use a 0.3 ml syringe.

Use needles of the right length and gauge (thickness). Shorter needles may be more comfortable but may not be suitable for overweight or obese people.

Insulin Pen Injectors

These look like thick pens; therefore, we refer to them commonly as insulin pens. There are two types of insulin pen injectors. The nondisposable type requires loading of the insulin cartridge or penfill into the pen. When the insulin runs out, a new cartridge of insulin is inserted. The disposable type, on the other hand, is preloaded with insulin and the entire pen injector is discarded when the insulin runs out. In both types, an injection needle has to be attached to it to deliver the insulin. The amount of insulin to be injected is set by a dialling or twisting mechanism.

Both types of insulin pens are more convenient as they do away with carrying separate syringes and insulin vials. With the insulin pens, smaller doses of insulin are more accurately administered. However, they cost more. Specific instructions are required for the various types of pen injectors.

Insulin Pump Devices

An insulin pump device, referred to simply as an insulin pump, is a small computerised device that can be programmed to deliver insulin continuously through a fine plastic tube inserted under the skin. It can also deliver boluses of insulin at meal times by pressing a few buttons. It is just a little larger than a pocket pager. Pump users have to monitor their blood sugars frequently to deliver the appropriate amount of bolus insulin. The insulin pump generally gives you better control and more meal flexibility, but it is a lot more costly and requires more frequent blood sugar monitoring. It is also more complex to use and requires more intensive learning. Some (more advanced models) have a wizard function that calculates for you the required pre-meal bolus insulin dose based on the amount of carbohydrate you are about to eat and the prevailing pre-meal blood glucose level.

Figure 9: An insulin pump can be worn discreetly under clothing while it delivers insulin.

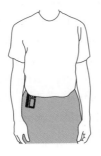
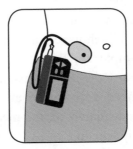

Inhaled Insulin

In 2006, both the American Food and Drug Administration (FDA) and the European Union approved the used of Exubera®, an inhalable insulin that was found to be effective in controlling blood sugar. This came in the form of a powder that was aerosolised and inhaled through the mouth using a special inhaler. The insulin used was a rapid or regular short-acting form. The onset of action of the inhaled insulin was relatively fast and therefore it had to be inhaled within 10 minutes before a meal. Type 1 diabetics took it in combination with a long-acting insulin. For Type 2 diabetes, it was used alone, with oral medications, or combined with a long-acting insulin. Post-marketing surveys were carried out to find out whether inhaled insulin was safe for smokers and people with chronic obstructive lung disease. Because of concern that it might increase the risk of lung cancer the marketing and further development of Exubera® was subsequently voluntarily halted by the manufacturer. In its wake, a new inhalable insulin, Afreeza® (Mannkind Corp.) is currently awaiting approval by the FDA. It is inhaled as a powder and absorbed into the blood stream. It apparently does not cause lung cancer in rats given a much higher dose than a human would normally be taking.

INSULIN REGIMENS

A person without diabetes has adequate insulin from the pancreas and does not have insulin resistance. His blood sugar is kept within a narrow normal range because there is a constant supply of basal insulin with automatic release of more insulin whenever blood glucose rises after a meal. Conversely, insulin will shut off automatically when blood sugar drops after prolonged fasting or during and after heavy exercise.

Insulin therapy seeks to mimic this physiological pattern but can never exactly achieve it, no matter how sophisticated the regimen is. The number of daily shots required varies from person to person. It is usually more complex for Type 1 diabetes than for Type 2 diabetes. In the former, because the lack of insulin is very extreme, at least twice daily shots are needed for control and survival. Type 2 diabetics who fail to respond adequately to oral medications may, initially, do well with a once-daily schedule.

Once injected, insulin remains in the body until it is degraded and cleared. There is no automatic shut off, hence the need to ensure that food intake matches the injected insulin to avoid hypoglycaemia.

Once-daily Insulin

In this regimen, a single daily shot of intermediate or long acting insulin is given, either in the morning or evening, to supplement any residual insulin the diabetic is still able to produce. This regimen works only if the pancreas is still able to contribute enough insulin with each meal, with or without the aid of oral diabetes medications. This regimen works only for Type 2 diabetes.

Twice- or Thrice-daily Insulin

This is the most common insulin regimen used in Type 1 diabetes, but some Type 2 diabetic patients may also eventually require such dosing. Three combinations are commonly used:

1. An intermediate-acting insulin only, given before breakfast and before dinner (this may be enough for Type 2 diabetes, but is usually not for Type 1 diabetes).
2. A combination of either regular (short-acting) or rapid-acting and intermediate-acting insulin before breakfast and before dinner.
3. Either of the regimens mentioned above plus either regular (short-acting) or rapid-acting insulin at lunchtime (that is, three injections a day).

Basal-bolus Regimen

Another more complex method uses a long-acting insulin given in the morning or late evening to provide basal insulin, plus either regular (short-acting) or rapid-acting insulin given at meal times to control the post-meal blood sugar surge. This means four injections a day if the patient takes three meals a day.

TIMING OF INSULIN INJECTIONS

The timing of insulin injections in relation to meals depends on the type of insulin. Regular (short-acting) insulin, either on its own or in combination with intermediate insulin, should be given about 30 to

45 minutes before meals. This ensures that the insulin is already in the bloodstream when the blood sugar rises after a meal. The exact timing of a regular (short-acting) insulin depends on the prevailing blood glucose, if it is known. The table below is a rough guide. If the pre-meal blood glucose is relatively low, inject nearer the meal. For example, the insulin is preferably injected 15 minutes before the meal if your blood glucose level is between 4.1–7 mmol/L, and 30 minutes if it is between 7.1–10 mmol/L.

Table 11: Timings of regular (short-acting) insulin injections

If blood sugar level before a meal is:	Inject insulin :
Below 3 mmol/L	When completing the meal
3.1 to 4 mmol/L	At meal time
4.1 to 7 mmol/L	15 minutes before the meal
7.1 to 10 mmol/L	30 minutes before the meal
Over 10 mmol/L	45 minutes before the meal

If in doubt, consult your diabetes care team.

Rapid-acting insulin (such as insulin lispro [Humalog®] and insulin aspart [Novorapid®]), used either singly or in combination with intermediate-acting insulin, should be injected 5 to 10 minutes before a meal since they are absorbed faster. Insulin glulisine or Apidra®, can be given just before or up to 20 minutes after a meal.

Insulin Glargine (Lantus®) and Insulin Detemir (Levemir®) do not have a peak action. Hence they need not be injected at any specific time before or after a meal but they are best injected at the same time each day, either in the morning or at night before bedtime. Although their action lasts about 24 hours, your doctor may instruct you to administer it twice a day to ensure better round-the-clock coverage.

INSULIN DOSE ADJUSTMENT

The starting insulin dose is empirically determined by your doctor and then adjusted according to the blood sugar response. Typically, the maintenance dose for adults is 0.5–1 unit per kg body weight per day for Type 1 diabetes and 0.3–1.5 units per kg per day for Type

2 diabetes. Your doctor will usually start at the lower end of the recommended dose and adjust the dose accordingly. Obese patients need more insulin to overcome their greater insulin resistance.

Even when you have settled to a fixed dose regimen, there will be times when you need to adjust your insulin dose, such as when you catch the flu, change your eating pattern or level of physical activity, and travel across time zones. In adults, changes in insulin dose adjustments are normally 1–2 units at a time, but can be 3–4 units for those who are overweight and more resistant to insulin.

Discuss the specific adjustments with your diabetes care team.

INJECTING INSULIN: TECHNIQUES AND SAFE HANDLING

When it comes to handling and injecting insulin, no amount of words, written or spoken, can do better than a good demonstration. The diabetes nurse clinician is your best bet on insulin injection without tears. This chapter will help you recall what you have learnt from the nurse. Injecting insulin need not be a nightmare if you resolve to do it right from the start.

Where to Inject Insulin

Insulin is injected subcutaneously, that is, under the skin where there is a layer of fat. From there, it is absorbed into the bloodstream and carried to its various sites of action.

The preferred injection site is usually based on convenience. The four main areas are the abdomen, the upper arm, the thigh and the buttocks. Your doctor or nurse will advise you on the best area to inject. Most people choose to inject into the abdominal wall.

Do not change your injection area frequently. This might cause excessive blood glucose swings. This happens because insulin moves into the bloodstream at different speeds from different areas—fastest when into the abdominal wall, followed by the arm and slowest when injected into the thigh or buttocks. It is better to use the same area regularly, but use a different spot within the same area each day.

Do not inject into the same spot repeatedly, although it is tempting to do so, as it becomes less painful after a while. Injecting into the same spot or small area repeatedly causes thickening of the layer below the skin—a condition called insulin lipohypertrophy. Insulin injected into these thickened sites may not be well absorbed. Changing your insulin injection *spot* will prevent this from happening. There should be enough area and you should use the same spot only once a month.

Before You Use Insulin

It is always a good habit to check the condition of the insulin and its expiry date before giving your insulin injection. Do not use it if:

- It has expired.
- There is any contamination or discoloration.
- There is floating debris in the insulin that does not dissolve when the bottle is rotated.
- A vial has been opened longer than a specified period (usually 4 to 6 weeks depending on the type and brand). Unexpected spoilage can occur, thus it is always good to have spare insulin available at all times.

How to Withdraw a Single Insulin Dose from a Vial

- Wash your hands with soap and water and dry them.
- Mix the insulin by slowly rolling the bottle between your hands. Never shake the bottle.
- Wipe the top of the vial with an alcohol swab.
- Be sure of the number of units of insulin you need to inject. Pull the plunger to draw in that amount of air into the syringe.
- Insert the needle into the upright vial of insulin and inject the air into the vial. With the needle still in the vial, hold up the vial upside down to eye level, then draw the required dose of insulin into the syringe.
- If there are air bubbles in the syringe, expel them back into the vial, but ensure that the correct number of units of insulin remains in the syringe.
- Remove the syringe (with the needle still fixed to it) from the vial.

How to Draw Out Two Types of Insulin into One Syringe

- Wash your hands with soap and water and dry them.
- Rotate the vial between your palms to mix the *cloudy* intermediate-acting insulin thoroughly.
- Inject the amount of air equal to the dose of insulin into the *cloudy* intermediate-acting insulin vial.
- Withdraw the needle from the vial.
- Draw in air equal to the dose of *clear* short-acting or rapid-acting insulin into the syringe, then inject the air into the *clear* regular insulin vial.
- Holding the vial upside down at eye level, draw the *clear* short-acting or rapid-acting insulin into the syringe to the required dose or marking.
- Insert the needle into the *cloudy* intermediate-acting insulin vial. Be careful not to push any *clear* insulin into the *cloudy* insulin. Holding the vial upside down, pull the plunger to draw out the correct dose of the *cloudy* insulin.
- At the end of the procedure, the amount of insulin in the syringe should be the total of *clear* and *cloudy* insulin.
- Remove the syringe (with the needle fixed to it) from the vial.

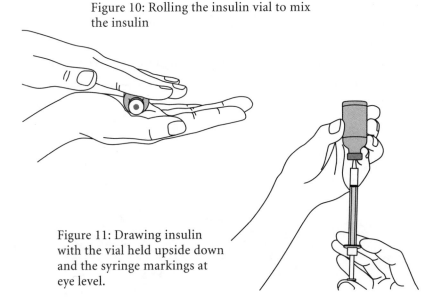

Figure 10: Rolling the insulin vial to mix the insulin

Figure 11: Drawing insulin with the vial held upside down and the syringe markings at eye level.

Note the following:
- *Clear* regular short-acting and rapid-acting insulin can be mixed with *cloudy* intermediate-acting insulin.
- Although insulin glargine (Lantus) is a long-acting insulin, it is also a clear solution, but it must not be mixed with other insulins.
- Always draw out the *clear* regular short-acting or rapid-acting insulin first during the mixing procedure.

Injecting Techniques
- The skin should be clean before injection. Cleansing with soap and water is preferred to alcohol or spirit because the latter tends to harden the skin.
- Gently pinch a fold of skin between your thumb and forefinger.
- Push the needle through the skin at a 90-degree angle, ensuring that the needle is inserted to its full length.
- It is best to use a 90-degree angle but, if you are thin, you may use an angle between 45 and 90 degrees.
- Push the plunger to inject the insulin, making sure that you inject all the insulin.
- Leave the needle in for several seconds.
- Pull the needle out at the same angle.
- Do not rub the injection site. Rubbing can disperse the insulin too quickly or cause irritation.
- Rotate injection spots to prevent the skin from thickening as this affects insulin absorption.

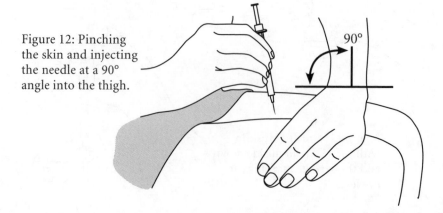

Figure 12: Pinching the skin and injecting the needle at a 90° angle into the thigh.

Figure 13: Pinching the skin and injecting the needle at a 45° angle into the abdomen, if you are thin.

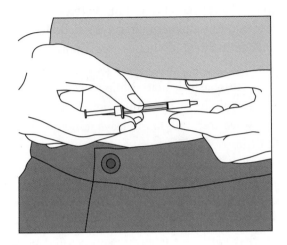

How to Make Injections More Comfortable

- Insulin at room temperature is preferred. Cold insulin straight from the refrigerator may hurt when injected.
- Ensure that there are no air bubbles in the syringe before you inject the insulin.
- Do not tense the muscles where you are giving the injection.
- Insert the needle with a quick jab. A hesitant slow action causes more discomfort.
- Pull the needle out at the same angle that it is plunged in.
- Use sharp needles. Yes, sharper needles are less painful or traumatic!

Injection Aids

If you have poor eyesight, you may need a syringe magnifier to help you see the markings on the vial and syringe barrel. Or you can use devices that aid in fixing the dose of insulin to be withdrawn. Other aids may have the needle hidden to make it less intimidating.

Storage of Insulin

Insulin makers advise storing your unopened insulin in the normal compartment of the refrigerator, not in the freezer. Also, keep it away from extreme heat. Extreme temperatures can destroy insulin.

As for the insulin currently being used, many users are under the wrong impression that it must always be kept in the fridge. This is not necessary as long as it is placed in a place that is not overheated or under direct sunlight or constant bright light. Therefore, keep it away from the stove area and do not leave it in your car if it is parked under the hot sun.

Insulin can be carried with you wherever you go, provided the above precautions are taken. Insulin vials/cartridges currently in use can be stored at room temperature for 4 to 6 weeks, depending on the type and brand. Cartridges in pen injectors and disposable pen injectors that you are currently using should be kept at room temperature to prevent clogging of the insulin.

When travelling, it is always a good practice to carry your insulin and syringes with you all the time. When flying, do not check in your insulin and accessories. Do not leave them in your car either, unless you do not need them for the time you are out of the car and the car is in a shaded area. In places where the weather can change quite quickly and unexpectedly (like in Melbourne), it is safer to take them out of the car.

Sharps Disposal

Sharps, such as syringes with attached needles, pen injector needles and lancets, are medical wastes that need to be disposed of correctly. The best way to dispose of sharps is to place them in a puncture-proof, heavy-duty plastic or metal container with a lid that can be sealed before disposal. If you do not dispose of your sharps properly, you could cause injury to yourself and others.

INCRETIN ANALOGUES

Incretin analogues are relatively new. They are an additional tool in the treatment of Type 2 diabetes, but not Type 1 diabetes. Although incretin analogues are not insulins and have some actions similar to some oral diabetes medications, they are injectables and, therefore, not included in the previous chapter.

An incretin analogue that is available in Singapore since mid 2008 is Exenatide (Byetta®). Another one that has just been approved by the US Food and Drug Administration (FDA) in January 2010 is Liraglutide (Victoza®).

Incretin analogues are modified incretins, hormones naturally found in the wall of the small intestines. A major incretin is glucagon-like peptide-1 or GLP-1 which lowers blood sugar through the following main mechanisms:

- Released when food is ingested, it stimulates the secretion of insulin and suppresses the secretion of glucagon from the pancreas.
- It slows down stomach emptying, causing food to take longer to pass from the stomach to the small intestines.
- It has actions on the brain to promote earlier satiety during a meal.

People with Type 2 diabetes, apart from being insulin resistant and insulin deficient, also produce less GLP-1 in response to a meal, compared to those without diabetes. Incretin analogues, therefore, fill the gap caused by this abnormality in the disease.

Clinical trials have confirmed that Exenatide, injected subcutaneously twice daily before meals, and Liraglutide, injected once a day, improve diabetes control. One of their advantages is that, unlike injected insulin, they do not cause weight gain and may even cause weight loss. Another advantage is that they stimulate the production and release of insulin only when the prevailing blood sugar is high, thus minimising the risk of hypoglycaemia, a potential hazard with insulin therapy and many oral diabetes medications. They have, therefore, been billed as 'intelligent' drugs.

Post-marketing surveillance of Exenatide has caused some concern that it might cause acute pancreatitis (inflammation of the pancreas), but the cause-effect relationship is far from proven.

In the pipeline is the development of longer acting incretin analogues that can be administered only once a week. If these prove to be efficacious, this would certainly be an advance.

04 WHAT IS GOOD CONTROL?

*"You can't hit a target you cannot see,
and you cannot see a target you do not have."*

—Hilary Hinton 'Zig' Ziglar (1926–)
American author, motivational coach and speaker

TARGETS OF CONTROL

Countless studies have confirmed that people with diabetes are healthier and have less complications if they maintain their blood glucose, blood pressure, weight and lipids within an established normal range. This is the reason why your diabetes care team keeps harping on these issues. Hence, it is vital that you know what the targets are and what your doctors and nurses are talking about.

Blood Glucose

Blood glucose, as you now know, are the buzz words. Your doctor is likely to test for it at every consultation. This may be a fasting blood glucose (after an overnight fast) or random blood glucose (done regardless of when the last meal was). The random blood glucose is particularly useful for assessing diabetes control if done one-and-a-half to two hours after a meal (postprandial or post-meal blood glucose). Use Table 12 to gauge how well you are doing.

Table 12: What your glucose levels mean[1]

Blood glucose (mmol/L)	Excellent	Good	Needs to be improved	Poor
Fasting (before meal)	4.0–6.0	6.1–8.0	8.1–10	more than 10
2 hours after a meal	5.0–7.0	7.1–10.0	10.1–13.0	more than 13

Excellent
Your glucose level is in the ideal range.

Good
Your glucose level is well controlled.

Needs to be improved
Glucose level is not very well controlled. Consult your doctor. This level of glucose, however, may be acceptable for certain groups of people, such as the elderly and those with advanced diabetic complications.

Poor
Your glucose level is unacceptable.

HbA1c

You will find that your doctor often does another blood test called HbA1c, short for haemoglobin A1c, at your periodic checkups. (For ease of communication, it is often further shortened to A1c.) It provides an indication of your average blood glucose over the previous two to three months. To understand the concept of this test, remember that haemoglobin (Hb) is the red pigment, found in the red blood cells, that carries oxygen to the tissues. Glucose and other forms of sugar get attached to it to form glycated haemoglobin. HbA1c is the major form of glycated haemoglobin.

The more glucose molecules there are in the blood, the more of them are attached to the Hb and the higher the HbA1c. In a non-diabetic person, HbA1c forms 4.5–6.4% of total Hb. This test gives an indication of the average blood glucose level over the last 2–3 months because this is the time period when Hb stays in the blood circulation before the red blood cells die. For this reason, the HbA1c test is usually done every three months (or longer if your diabetes is stable).

HbA1c Targets and Interpreting the HbA1c Test

The following HbA1c targets have been adopted:

Table 13: HbA1c targets[2]

HbA1c levels (%)	Diabetes control
4.5–6.4	Ideal (Excellent)
6.5–7.0	Optimal (Good)
7.1–8.0	Suboptimal (Needs improvement)
> 8.0	Unacceptable (Poor)

As an illustration, if your HbA1c level is 8%, your diabetes control is unacceptable. Remember, however, that an HbA1c of 8% is not equal to a blood glucose of 8 mmol/L. Instead, it is equivalent to about 11.5 mmol/L, as shown in the following table. On the other hand, if your HbA1c level is 6%, you are in optimal control.

Table 14: Correlation between HbA1c levels and mean plasma glucose[3]

HbA1c	Plasma glucose* (mmol/L)	Plasma glucose* (mg/dL)
6%	7.5	135
7%	9.5	170
8%	11.5	205
9%	13.5	240
10%	15.5	275
11%	17.5	310
12%	19.5	345

*Plasma glucose is generally slightly higher than whole blood glucose.

The HbA1c test does not have to be done after an overnight fast. Unlike the blood glucose test, it is not a reflection of what you have just eaten. It is important to stress this point because, time and again, whenever we inform a patient of his high HbA1c, he would explain that he had just eaten a big meal. On the contrary, the HbA1c is a window to the blood glucose level of the last three months!

Therefore, do look back at the last three months to find out what has gone wrong. It does not mean it is entirely your fault (overeating, not exercising enough or not taking your medications). It simply means that you and your doctor or diabetes nurse or dietitian need to see what could have gone wrong and what can be done. It may mean a need to step up medication dosage or change medications.

If you have a consistent HbA1c of less than 6.6–7%, you lower your risk of chronic diabetic complications. However, the risk of hypoglycaemia may be increased when you aim for a perfect HbA1c.

Having a consistently normal HbA1c is not all there is to it. HbA1c, being an index of average blood glucose, can be within the normal range if there has been more or less equal numbers of low and high blood glucose levels over the last three months. Therefore, you should aim for a good or excellent HbA1c value and periodic self-monitored blood glucose levels that are as near normal as possible, without wild swings between high and low readings (refer to Tables 12 and 13 above).

Under certain circumstances, your target glycaemic control (in terms of HbA1c and periodic blood glucose) may not be very stringent. Your doctor will have to consider your age, life expectancy, presence of complications and other medical conditions, your proneness to hypoglycaemia and home circumstances. Remember that the whole aim of achieving good control is to alleviate symptoms, prevent acute and chronic complications and promote overall quality of life. When advanced chronic complications have already developed, 'the boat has been missed', as it were. If the patient is already elderly, chronic complications are less likely to develop since it takes a longer period of poor control to develop these complications. The priority in this case is to relieve symptoms and prevent acute complications (like infection, diabetic ketoacidosis and hyperosmolar hyperglycaemia syndrome) and this can be achieved without having to aim for perfect blood glucose levels.

Blood Lipids (Cholesterol and Triglyceride)

People with diabetes often have abnormal blood lipid (fats) levels. These usually take the form of high triglyceride and low high-density-lipoprotein cholesterol (HDL cholesterol, the so-called 'good' cholesterol). The total cholesterol and low-density-lipoprotein cholesterol (LDL cholesterol, the so-called 'bad' cholesterol) may also be high. This combination increases the risk of heart attacks, strokes and foot gangrene.

You should, therefore, have your blood lipids checked regularly. If the levels are not on target, and if regular exercise and dietary measures are not adequate to improve the profile, you will need to take medication.

Table 15: Lipid targets for people with diabetes[4]

LDL cholesterol ('bad' cholesterol)	Less than 2.6 mmol/L*
Triglycerides	Less than 1.7 mmol/L
HDL cholesterol ('good' cholesterol)	More than 1.0 mmol/L

*In high-risk individuals, an LDL-cholesterol target of less than 2 mmol/L may be necessary to protect the heart.

Blood Pressure

The ideal blood pressure target for a person with diabetes is more stringent (that is, lower) than that for someone without diabetes. It is internationally accepted, based on research data, that this target should be 130/80 mmHg or below.

Weight

Maintaining an ideal body weight (BMI 18.5–22.9 kg/m^2) has lots of benefits for the overweight person at risk of diabetes or already with diabetes. Suffice to say it prevents diabetes and helps control blood glucose and blood pressure. Weight reduction, sometimes, is all that is required to achieve the desired glucose, blood pressure and lipid targets as discussed in previous chapters.

WHEN THE GOING IS GOOD, KEEP GOING

Unfortunately, doctors have not found a cure for diabetes yet. What we are doing is merely containing the situation. When you have hit the appropriate target, you have to maintain it for as long as you can. The stark reality is that dietary measures and physical activity should always not be let up. It is good to have a reward system to keep you going but consider a new dress, a spa treatment, a concert or a healthy meal instead of unhealthy 'treats'.

Case 11: Mdm SKM – Unhealthy Reward (Find a Better Alternative)

Middle-aged SKM, who has had diabetes for 10 years, managed to achieve a HbA1c of 7% and an LDL-cholesterol of 2.45 mmol/L, only to see the figures climb to 8.4% and 3.39 mmol/L, respectively, over five months. While exploring the possible causes why control had faltered after the initial success, she readily admitted that she "rewarded herself" by slacking on her diet when she was getting acceptable sugar readings.

05 MONITORING DIABETES CONTROL

"I am only one, but still I am one. I cannot do
everything, but still I can do something; and because
I cannot do everything, I will not refuse
to do something I can do."

—Edward Everett Hale (1822–1909)
American author and clergyman

SELF-BLOOD GLUCOSE MONITORING (SBGM)

Monitoring your blood glucose is so important and such an integral part of good diabetes management that we are devoting a whole chapter to it. We call it self-blood glucose monitoring or SBGM.

While the HbA1c is extremely useful in telling you the average blood sugar over the last three months (see Chapter 4), it does not help you get a handle on day-to-day management. The introduction of portable glucose meters (or glucometers) more than 20 years ago has revolutionised the way diabetes is managed. Without it, you and your diabetes care team would not have a precise feel of what the day-to-day blood sugar is. SBGM is sometimes also written as SMBG (self-monitoring of blood glucose or self-monitored blood glucose).

With very few exceptions, all diabetics find it a dread to do SBGM because of the need to prick the finger to get a drop of blood, even if the finger pricking is done by a family member. Some will absolutely not do it, some cannot do it because of disabilities, while others find it a financial burden. Very few actually overdo it. See Figures 14 and 15.

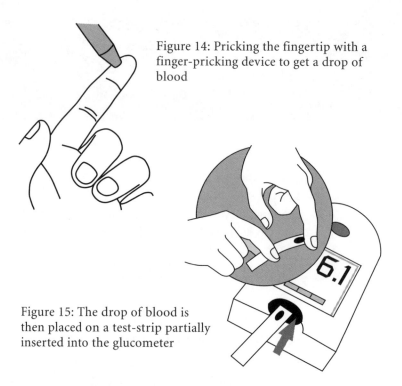

Figure 14: Pricking the fingertip with a finger-pricking device to get a drop of blood

Figure 15: The drop of blood is then placed on a test-strip partially inserted into the glucometer

There are many glucometers available. Some common blood glucose meters are Advantage, Glucometer Elite, Precision, Sure Step, Optium and Smart Scan.

Benefits of SBGM

There are several benefits of SBGM. It complements the HbA1c that is usually done every 3 to 6 months.

By giving you the blood sugar reading at a point in time, it helps you see the relationship between food eaten, physical activity and diabetes medications taken, especially if there has been a recent change in your usual routine. You will thus be able to make immediate changes to your diet in response to blood sugar levels that are either consistently too high or too low.

For instance, if your blood sugar before lunch is always high, it may be because of excessive carbohydrates in your breakfast or mid-morning snack or a reduction of your usual morning physical activities. Remember that you may feel perfectly well even though your blood sugar is high. Conversely, the blood glucose may be consistently too low. This will alert you to adjust your meal size and activities accordingly. Any abnormally high or low reading may also alert your doctor to modify your medications.

It enables you to know whether symptoms you encounter (such as blurring of vision, palpitations, lapses in memory, etc.) are due to extremes of blood sugar level. This will alert you to either impending diabetic ketoacidosis (DKA), or hyperosmolar hyperglycaemia syndrome (HHS) (see Chapter 2) or hypoglycaemia (see Chapters 2 and 6).

How Often and When to Do SBGM

There are no hard and fast rules. A lot depends on the prevailing situation. Your doctor or nurse will give you general or specific guidelines. Remember, the more often you check your blood glucose the more you will understand your diabetes. For example, stable diabetics need to do SBGM less often than those who have just been diagnosed and have just started treatment or had their treatment changed. More on this below.

The intensity of self-tests may take one of several formats:

1. Two-point Test

Test pre-breakfast and post-meal. Spread out the post-meal tests to include post-breakfast, post-lunch and post-dinner. This way, you will get a spread-out picture of your blood glucose.

This is recommended for stable Type 2 diabetics and those on one or two insulin injections daily, who are unable to do more frequent checks.

2. Four-point Test

Test pre-meal before each of the three main meals and at bedtime. This is often recommended for those on twice daily insulin injections and those whose diabetes treatment is being altered. For the latter, this is the minimum number of times to allow adjustments of insulin dose. The four-point tests can be done daily or on alternate days depending on circumstances.

3. Seven-point Test

Test pre-meal (before each main meal) and post-meal (after each main meal) and at bedtime. This is often recommended for women with diabetes during pregnancy, those who have just started intensive insulin therapy (four injections a day) or those using the insulin pump and who need to make fine adjustments to the insulin dosage. Again, this can be done daily or two to three days a week, depending on individual circumstances and inclination.

Note on terminology: Pre-meal refers to the time immediately before a meal and post-meal refers to 2 hours ± 30 minutes after the start of a meal. Bedtime tests, conventionally, refer to 10 pm–12 midnight, even if you go to bed past midnight.

When Extra Tests Are Recommended

Outside of a recommended routine schedule, extra tests should be done under certain circumstances, such as:

- Before and after exercise.
- When you suspect hypoglycaemia. You may need to do a check in the middle of the night (between 2 and 4 am) if nocturnal hypoglycaemia is suspected.
- When you are developing unawareness to hypoglycaemia (more on this in Chapter 6). You should be alerted to it when your routine test shows low readings and yet there are no warning symptoms.
- When you have symptoms that might suggest high blood glucose. Remember that nausea, vomiting and abdominal pain may be signs of very high glucose levels and impending diabetic ketoacidosis (DKA) (see Chapter 2).
- During conditions of stress, e.g. infection, injury, pregnancy, menstruation or even examinations.
- When you are making changes to your food and activity routine and to your medications, especially insulin.
- When you have lost weight or gained weight.
- When you are on intensive insulin treatment (three or four insulin injections per day).

- During the week or two before a routine clinic visit. More frequent tests will enable your diabetes care team to adjust your treatment more precisely, if necessary.

Proper SBGM Technique and Accurate Records

SBGM is to help you and your diabetes care team understand and optimise your diabetes control. Doing it properly and keeping clear and accurate records are vital for correct interpretation of the results. Bring along the readings during each visit to the doctor or to your diabetes nurse.

The memory in the glucometer is a wonderful function for recalling the results, but it is easier and less time-consuming to study the glucose pattern on a hard copy record than having to scroll up and down for the results stored in the meter.

Never share your glucometer with someone else, as his or her blood glucose records will remain in the meter's memory, causing confusion. Furthermore, there is the risk of contamination with someone else's blood. If you must share the use of a glucometer, ensure that you exclude the other person's blood glucose results from your hard copy record.

The following cases below emphasise the importance of doing SBGM correctly and keeping accurate records.

Case 12: Mr MRE – Calibrating Your Glucose Meter

Mr MRE, aged 66 years, was on insulin therapy. He tested his blood glucose religiously at home. Results ranged from 10 mmol/L to 12.7 mmol/L at different times of the day and he was disappointed. However, his HbA1c was between 5% and 6% on two consecutive months. There was nothing (such as anaemia) that could have falsely lowered the HbA1c. He had not suffered any periods of low blood glucose (hypoglycaemia). His doctor was initially puzzled, but a quick check of his glucometer showed that he did not calibrate his glucometer when he bought new test strips. The problem was rectified, and the next time he saw his doctor, the home blood glucose readings he presented ranged from 6.2–8.5 mmol/L, consistent with an HbA1c reading of 6.8% and indicating excellent control of his diabetes. He was happy, and so was his doctor. His doctor was able to reduce his insulin dose a little.

Case 13: Mr TS – Falsifying Blood Glucose Records. (Don't Ever!)

Mr TS, currently 54 years old, has had diabetes since the age of 33, and was taking insulin twice a day. There was a time in 1998 when his doctor was puzzled over his high HbA1c of 10.3% when his self-monitored blood glucose (SMBG) readings kept showing between 5.2 to 9.5 mmol/L. If this were indeed the pattern, his HbA1c should be about 8%, not 10.3%. Either his glucometer was faulty or he was not doing the test correctly. The diabetes nurse educator found no fault with the meter or his technique. Mr TS later confessed that he had falsified the readings because he wanted to show his doctor that everything was all right. The memory in the meter showed that the blood glucose range over the same period was actually between 9.3 and 12.8 mmol/L. He felt bad about it but it was good that he admitted to the falsification. His doctor then added metformin to his treatment on the basis that it was actually in poor control. His HbA1c subsequently improved to 7.8% and 7.1% over the next three and five months respectively.

Figure 16: A patient's self-monitored blood glucose records

Ms C.T.

Day										
Date		1/12	5/12	10/12	18/12	26/12	2/01	8/01	13/01	22/01
Breakfast	: Before*	6·00			9·1	5·8		7·8		8·1
	: 2 hours after			8·7			6·1		9·7	
Lunch	: Before*		8·1		6·5			7·1		10·8
	: 2 hours after					8·0	11·5		10·1	
Dinner	: Before*	7·00			10·2	9·7				9·7
	: 2 hours after		9·2				12·1	8·6		
Bedtime	: > 3 hours after dinner									
	: Middle of the night									
Hypoglycaemic symptoms										
Insulin dose :										
Tablet dose :										
Comments:										
Diet										
Activity										

Note: Tests are done at different times of the day in relation to meal times, providing adequate information to evaluate control.

CONTINUOUS GLUCOSE MONITORING SYSTEM (CGMS)

Several companies have developed the CGMS for more precise and complete tracking of blood glucose. A sensor inserted under the skin measures glucose in the fluid around tissues (called interstitial fluid) every five minutes over three days. The glucose level in the interstitial fluid correlates very well with that in the blood.

The data, picked up wirelessly by a small receiver worn by the user, is then downloaded onto a computer for analysis using a special programme, to give the blood glucose pattern. By relating the blood glucose tracing to meals, physical activity and medications, you get a better understanding of your blood sugar trend. Compared to self-monitored blood glucose, which gives you only snapshots of your blood glucose, the CGMS tells you what your blood glucose is in between these snapshots and how fast it is changing.

In more advanced versions of the CGMS, blood glucose data is wirelessly transmitted from the sensor/transmitter to a small receiver or monitor worn on the user to give real-time recordings, complete with alerts of preset low or high levels and glucose direction trends.

Your doctor may use the CGMS on you to supplement self-blood glucose monitoring (SBGM) if the latter is unable to solve problems of glycaemic control. See Graph 3.

SUPPLEMENTARY TEST—URINE KETONE TEST

Monitoring the state of your diabetes control should include doing a urine test for ketones, when indicated.

The presence of ketones, when your blood glucose is high, may herald the onset of diabetic ketoacidosis (DKA) (see Chapter 2). Therefore, you should check your urine for ketones if your blood glucose hits above 15 mmol/L or 300 mg/dL. Note that the urine ketones may test positive after a prolonged fast. In this situation, your blood glucose is low, rather than high, and its presence in this situation is, therefore, not serious. Commercially available urine ketone test strips include Gluketur and Labstix.

Graph 3: Continuous glucose monitoring of a patient on insulin treatment.

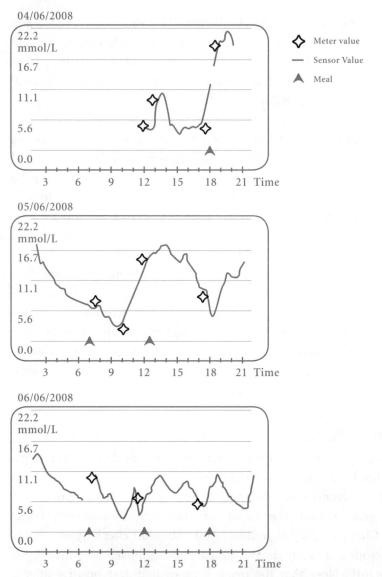

04/06/2008

05/06/2008

06/06/2008

Note: This patient's blood glucose was clearly high after dinner on the first day and for 2–3 hours before lunch on the second day, but, by making alterations to his meals, the blood glucose levels throughout the day were much improved on the third day.

SBGM—AN OPTION AND A BANE?

If you are still hesitant about doing SBGM or find it a chore, consider that current glucose meters have improved in the last two decades— they are smaller, give faster results, and the lancing devices have spring-loaded lancets that are hidden from view. Many companies are working on developing minimally or non-invasive instruments that can measure blood glucose without using a drop of blood. In the meantime, use SBGM to help you control your blood glucose better, as you look forward to the day when new innovations will be available to you.

06 HYPOGLYCAEMIA

"Chance favours the prepared mind."

—Louis Pasteur (1822–1895)
French chemist and biologist.

HYPOGLYCAEMIA AND DIABETES

Hypoglycaemia occurs when the blood glucose falls to a level at which the cells of the body, including the brain cells, do not get adequate glucose to function.Why are we talking about low blood sugar or hypoglycaemia? Is not diabetes all about high blood glucose or sugar? The reality is that hypoglycaemia (often shortened to 'hypo' for ease of communication) is, indeed, a problem in diabetes.

How is this so? Remember what we said earlier in Chapter 1. A person without diabetes is able to switch insulin on and off quickly depending on whether the prevailing blood sugar is high or low, thus keeping it within a normal range (between 4 and 8 mmol/L). The person with diabetes, on the other hand, is attempting to control his blood sugar with either tablets or insulin or both. This is rather non-physiological and does not mimic exactly the actual situation in someone without diabetes. Insulin, once stimulated by tablets or injected into the body, does not switch off when the blood sugar drops to a level that normally switches it off, hence the development of 'hypo' (below 3.5 mmol/L).

Causes of Hypoglycaemia
- Eating too little carbohydrates or not eating after taking your medication
- Excessive exercise without eating enough food
- Excessive doses of insulin and/or diabetes tablets

- Illnesses, especially when appetite is poor
- Incorrect timing of insulin or anti-diabetes tablets in relation to meals
- Taking alcohol without taking food
- Interference by other medications that enhance the actions of diabetes medications

Signs and Symptoms of Hypoglycaemia
- Tiredness and weakness
- Trembling
- Hunger
- Palpitations (a sensation of fast heart beat)
- Sweating
- Dizziness or headache
- Sensation of pins and needles around lips and mouth

With more severe hypoglycaemia (below 3 mmol/L), you may also experience:
- Confusion/inability to do simple tasks
- Behavioural changes
- Slurred speech
- Drowsiness
- Unconsciousness

You should inform your family and people whom you are in daily contact with about these warning signs, so that they can help you deal with the 'hypos', should they occur.

Remember that many of these symptoms may be due to other causes, such as sheer anxiety or even impending stroke. When in doubt, check your blood glucose.

Nocturnal Hypoglycaemia
'Hypos' can occur at any time of day. When it occurs in the middle of the night while you are sleeping, it is called a 'nocturnal hypo'. Usually, you will be awakened by restless sleep and even nightmares, drenched in sweat. At other times, you may sleep right through a 'hypo' and the only indication is finding that your pyjamas and bedsheet are soaked

when you wake up. The person sleeping next to you should be aware that your restless tossing around and thrashing about in bed may not be due to an ordinary bad dream but may be a sign of a 'hypo'. He or she needs to know about this potential problem.

When nocturnal hypos occur frequently, test your blood sugar before you go to bed and at about 2 or 3 am for a few nights. Try, also, to recall the previous day's events, such as food intake, physical activities and medication. This will help you identify the cause of the hypoglycaemia. A bedtime carbohydrate snack may have to be taken routinely to prevent recurring nocturnal hypos.

Ways to Prevent Hypoglycaemia

- Proper timing of meals and medications is important. Frequent blood glucose tests after meals will help you find the right match.
- Take extra food before and after intensive exercise. You may even have to take a snack during a prolonged activity. Monitor your blood glucose after the exercise (see Chapter 3, Part 3).
- Do not consume alcohol on an empty stomach. When drinking alcohol, be sure to take some carbohydrate-containing foods at the same time. Be vigilant after alcohol consumption as excessive alcohol in your body makes it more difficult for the liver to produce glucose in response to 'hypos'.

What To Do During a 'Hypo'

1. If you are able to, confirm that you have a 'hypo' by testing your blood sugar.
2. If your blood sugar level is low, take 15–20 g of a carbohydrate snack immediately. Pure glucose would be best but, if it is not available, any form of carbohydrate would do, if eaten immediately. (See examples in the box.)
3. Rest. If you do not feel better after 10 to 15 minutes, take another portion of the glucose or carbohydrate. If your blood sugar level is still low after that, seek medical attention.
4. When you recover, eat a snack, e.g. cheese, crackers or your regular meal to prevent recurrence of the 'hypo'. Extra food taken to treat the 'hypo' is not counted as part of your usual

diet, so do not eat less food later in the day to compensate. Bring forward the next meal if hypoglycaemia occurs within half an hour of the meal.

5. Check with your doctor about the need to change your treatment if you experience frequent 'hypos'.

As 'hypos' can be very distressing, many patients tend to over-react and over-treat, resulting in subsequent high blood glucose. Therefore, check your blood sugar over the next few hours when you have fully recovered. With experience, you will, hopefully, avoid over-treatment. As many of the 'hypo' symptoms may be due to other causes, to avoid unnecessary treatment with glucose, check your blood glucose whenever you are not sure.

Some examples of fast-acting sugar sources
- A half glass of fruit juice
- 2 to 4 teaspoons of sugar, honey or syrup
- 1 glass of milk
- 3 glucose sweets (e.g. B-D glucose tablets)
- 5 sugar cubes or sweets (not sugar-free)
- 1 small box of raisins

Note:
- Liquid carbohydrates and sugars act faster than solid forms. Glucose acts faster than ordinary sugar.
- Do not use diabetic or low-calorie drinks or snacks to treat hypoglycaemia. They do not contain actual or adequate glucose.
- If you have taken the anti-diabetes medication acarbose (Glucobay®) in the last few hours, you will need to take only glucose to reverse the hypoglycaemia. Complex carbohydrates may not be effective, as their digestion is hindered by the acarbose still present in your gastrointestinal tract. (For more information on acarbose, see Chapter 3, Part 4.)

When Hypoglycaemia Leads to Unconsciousness

This advice is for people who live and work with the diabetic person (family members and colleagues).

1. Do not give the unconscious person any food or drink.
2. Roll the person onto his/her side.
3. Inject 1 mg glucagon into the arm or leg muscle. The glucagon should take effect in 15 to 20 minutes. An intravenous injection of 25–50 ml of 50% dextrose solution is the most effective way to raise the blood glucose. Take this action only if you absolutely know how to use these items. Otherwise,
4. Call for an ambulance (995).

Hypoglycaemia Unawareness

Some diabetic people may not have the usual warning signs and symptoms of hypoglycaemia. They may lose consciousness without warning. This condition is called hypoglycaemia unawareness and more commonly affect the elderly, those who have recurrent episodes of 'hypo', those who have had diabetes for a long time, and those with autonomic neuropathy (see Chapter 2). You may also not be aware of impending hypoglycaemia if you are taking medications that mask the usual symptoms, for example beta-blockers used for treating hypertension and coronary heart disease.

You can suspect you have this problem if, during a routine blood glucose test, you hit a low value and yet feel normal; if you wake up in the morning drenched in sweat but seemed to have slept right through; or when people around you notice you act 'funny' or are incoherent or confused but you did not have some of the warning symptoms mentioned earlier. If you are in this situation, do more routine blood glucose checks and before driving, swimming or any other activity that might put you and/or others in danger. You should also test between 2 am and 4 am if nocturnal 'hypo' is suspected. Work with your diabetes care team on this matter. Changing your medications, especially your insulin schedule, may be indicated.

Case 14: Mdm KBM – Hypoglycaemia because of Late Breakfast and No Dinner

Mdm KBM, who has had diabetes for 10 years, said that she was generally well, except for feeling dizzy and an intense hunger in the morning and around 2 am on a few occasions. Although she knew the rules, she had broken them on those occasions. She took her breakfast an hour and a half after her morning insulin injection because she wanted to have breakfast at work rather than at home. This caused the hypo as, by then, her insulin had started to act before she had time to take her breakfast. The nocturnal hypo was because she "did not feel like eating her dinner" even though she had already administered her pre-dinner insulin.

Comments: Even if you know that you can usually get to your place of work for breakfast in good time, you cannot anticipate when you will be caught in a traffic jam. If you really must do what Mdm KBM did, estimate the travelling time and keep some sugar on you for emergencies. Although diabetics are always reminded to watch their diet, skipping dinner after having taken insulin is not what 'watching your diet' means.

Case 15: Mr SG – Nocturnal 'Hypo' because of Excessive Exercise

Mr SG, who was 53 years old, had diabetes for four years and was taking gliblenclamide (5 mg in the morning and 2.5 mg at dinner time) and metformin (250 mg twice daily). He was doing fairly well with a HbA1c of 7.6%. His exercise routine was usually 30 to 45 minutes of brisk walking prior to dinner. One day, he decided to exercise after dinner and for 90 minutes. That night, he developed hypo in the middle of the night with palpitations and cold sweat. The symptoms were relieved by taking bread and Milo.

Comments: An increase in the level of physical activity can certainly lead to 'hypo'. To prevent it, you should take extra carbohydrates after the activity and ensure that at bedtime, your blood glucose is at least 5 mmol/L.

Case 16: Mr TYM – Insufficient Breakfast /Hypoglycaemia Unawareness

In one of his clinic visits, five months after starting insulin, 76-year-old Mr TYM (see Case 10, Chapter 3 Part 5) had a blood glucose of 2.0 mmol/L, which was clearly low, but he had no symptoms of hypoglycaemia. After taking an apple, his blood glucose was still 2.1 mmol/L. It turned out that that morning, he had taken his morning insulin as usual at 6.30 am and had less than his usual breakfast—two slices of plain bread, a hard-boiled egg and plain water. Mr TYM also revealed that his home blood glucose would usually be about 10 mmol/L one hour after his usual 'normal' breakfast.

Comments: Two important lessons can be learnt from this case. The first is that blood sugar is very dependent on the food we eat, in particular the carbohydrate portions. In this case, all the carbohydrates came from the bread and that was clearly not enough for Mr TYM (although it may be enough for others). The second lesson is that hypoglycaemia may not produce any symptoms, especially in longstanding diabetes and in older people. Hence, the importance of periodic self-checking of blood glucose to detect unsuspected low blood sugar. If it escapes detection and drops further, it may be disastrous. In the case of Mr TYM, the situation also called for a reduction in the total insulin dosage, which was duly done, as the incident happened while he was waiting to see his doctor.

Case 17: Mr HPL – Hypoglycaemia Coma because of Delaying Lunch

Mr HPL is a Type 1 diabetic on insulin. One Sunday, he was out with his family and it was time for lunch. Because he did not like what was on the menu, he decided to go home instead. Soon after he reached home, he passed out from a severe hypoglycaemic attack. Luckily, another son was at home and he was revived by intravenous glucose after the emergency ambulance service was called in.

Comments: Do not delay meals if you are on regular insulin injections. Losing consciousness from hypoglycaemia should, at all costs, be avoided.

Case 18: Ms LP – Nocturnal Hypolycaemia? Speak to Your Diabetes Team

Ms LP was full of zest when she first started work. She had just graduated from university. She had had Type 1 diabetes for 10 years. Her diabetes control had only been fair all this while. Now that she had just started work, she decided to improve her diabetes control. She started jogging after dinner several times a week and only took a bedtime snack if she felt hungry. She soon started experiencing severe low blood sugar in the early hours of the morning during her sleep. Her mother even had to force some sugary food into her mouth. She felt miserable and upset. LP then remembered that her diabetes care team was just a telephone call away. She was advised to check her blood sugar at bedtime and to take a bedtime snack, especially if she exercised in the evenings. She also took her intermediate-acting insulin just before bedtime, instead of before dinner, and seldom had nocturnal hypos thereafter.

Comments: LP took appropriate measures. Shifting the intermediate-action insulin to late evening delays the peak action of the insulin to nearer breakfast time, by which time LP would have woken up.

SMART MOVE

If you have a lot of 'hypos', bring them up with your diabetes care team to find out the cause and to review your treatment. Do some preliminary investigations on your own, such as monitoring your food intake and blood sugar, then go prepared with a clear description of the events.

07 MANAGING DIABETES DURING AN ACUTE ILLNESS

"Our greatest glory is not in never falling,
but in rising every time we fall."

—*Confucius (551–479 BCE)*
Chinese philosopher

Acute illnesses (such as a common flu, an injury, a heart attack, pneumonia, or surgery) are all stressors to the body that will cause the adrenals to release stress hormones. These stress hormones raise blood sugar by countering the actions of insulin. Hitherto stable blood sugar levels can quickly spin out of control.

Antibiotic and cough syrups are often, mistakenly, blamed for making diabetes worse during an illness. However, a dose of antibiotic or cough syrup contains only about 5 g of sugar and is not going to make a lot of difference to blood sugar levels. It is the illness itself that is to blame. On the other hand, if your appetite is severely reduced because of the illness, your blood sugar may fall.

GUIDELINES

It is important to follow the guidelines in this chapter so that your diabetes stays on course. If you are not sure what to do, contact your diabetes care team.

Do Not Skip Meals

Continue with your usual meal plan as closely as possible, but be prepared to modify it according to how you feel and what foods you can tolerate.

If you are unable to take your regular meals, replace them with alternatives. Examples include the following:

- Six level tablespoons of Ensure or Glucerna mixed with water
- One glass of milk with four cream crackers
- Six level teaspoons of malted milk powder or cocoa (e.g. Horlicks, Milo/Ovaltine) mixed with one glass of milk
- One and a half medium-size Chinese rice bowl of porridge with minced meat, chicken or fish
- Macaroni or *kway teow* (flat rice noodles) soup

If you are vomiting or have diarrhoea, drink plenty of fluids to prevent dehydration. If you cannot retain any food or fluids, consult your diabetes care team immediately.

Return to your usual meal plan as your symptoms subside and your appetite returns to normal.

Monitor Blood Sugar and Urine Ketones

Test your blood sugar more often and record all the results. You may need to do this every 2 to 4 hours. If the blood sugar is persistently more than 15 mmol/L for Type 1 diabetes, or more than 17 mmol/L for Type 2 diabetes, extra insulin or supplementary insulin is needed.

In addition to checking blood sugar, do a urine ketones test whenever the blood glucose is above 15 mmol/L. The presence of ketones in the urine is a warning of impending diabetic ketoacidosis (DKA) and the blood sugar should be quickly lowered. If you are not sure what you should do with a high blood sugar and positive urine ketones test, consult your diabetes care team.

Continue Taking Your Diabetes Medications

- Unless otherwise directed, take your usual dose of insulin and diabetes tablets even if you are not eating your *usual* diet.
- You may need to adjust the doses (e.g. inject more rapid or regular short-acting insulin) based on blood sugar readings.
- If you are on oral diabetes medication, you may temporarily require insulin to control your blood sugar.

Rest

Do not exercise but have more rest. Do not ever think you can 'try to sweat it out'. Physical activity during a flu can harm your heart. It will also destabilise your blood sugar and make it harder to control.

See Your Doctor if You Have Been:
- Sick for more than one day without improvement.
- Vomiting and having diarrhoea for more than 6 hours.
- Getting positive urine ketones tests.
- Getting persistently high blood sugars of more than 15 mmol/L.

Case 19: Mr KSH – Worsening of Diabetes Control during a Flu

Forty-year-old Mr KSH reluctantly accepted an increase in his diabetes medicine by his doctor who had noticed a gradual worsening of his sugar control over the last one year. A few weeks later, he contracted the flu and reduced his diabetes medicine for a few days, as he was not eating well. He skipped it entirely one morning and felt even more sick. Fortunately, he checked his blood sugar and got a fright when it showed a reading of 19.1 mmol/L. He quickly rang his doctor who told him not to stop his diabetes medication, advice he wisely followed. He resumed his diabetes medicine and as the flu got better, so did the blood sugar. He was not in the habit of doing frequent glucose tests but this time he remembered his doctor's advice and got the situation under control.

Comments: The lesson is that while a flu can take away your appetite, the stress on the body can still tip the balance towards a net rise in your blood sugar. Therefore, check your blood glucose frequently. Unless it is low, you should continue to take your diabetes medicine.

"Being defeated is often a temporary condition.
Giving up is what makes it permanent."

—*Marilyn vos Savant (1946–)*
American author, playwright, columnist and lecturer

THE SPECTRUM OF DIABETIC EYE DISEASE

Diabetes mellitus is the commonest cause of blindness in developing and developed countries. It causes diabetic retinopathy, macular oedema, cataract and glaucoma. Although, in most cases, vision can be restored, improved or stabilised with modern treatment, prevention is still better than cure.

Diabetic retinopathy refers to damage to the retina, the innermost layer of the eyeball, where images are formed and transmitted by nerves to the brain. Diabetic retinopathy often co-exists with macular oedema. Macular oedema is a condition in which the macula (the most light-sensitive part of the retina) is swollen, due to leakage of fluid from fragile retinal blood vessels.

Diabetic retinopathy declares itself in several ways. The earliest changes are out-pouchings (microaneurysms) of the weakened capillaries, showing up as tiny red dots. Patches of dot and blot haemorrhages on the retina may also appear at this stage. Clear sharp yellow patches (hard exudates) on the retina represent scars from such haemorrhages (see Figure 18). As the condition worsens, the retinal capillaries begin to clamp down. This leads to the appearance of soft, light yellow 'cotton wool' exudates, which represent damage to the nerve structures from lack of blood supply. Capillary closure also leads to formation of new but fragile vessels (neovascularisation). These new vessels may bleed more extensively into the vitreous humour behind the eye lens, giving rise to vitreous haemorrhage. In time, this vitreous haemorrhage forms fibrous tissues which can pull the retina layer forward, causing retinal detachment.

Diabetic retinopathy and macular oedema are conditions you see only in diabetes. Longstanding, poorly controlled diabetes, high blood pressure, high cholesterol levels, presence of protein in the urine (diabetic nephropathy), anaemia and smoking are risk factors for diabetic retinopathy. All these factors must be corrected to protect the retina. Pregnancy is also a risk factor.

Although cataract and glaucoma also occur in the general population, they occur more frequently and at an earlier age in diabetes. Cataracts are caused by the cloudiness of the eye lens as an indirect result of higher levels of glucose in the lens. Glaucoma is a condition in which the pressure in the space in front of the eye lens is increased. It may cause pain, eye redness and blurring of vision.

Figure 17: Normal retina

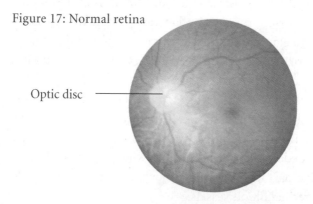

Optic disc

Figure 18: Diabetic retinopathy showing hard exudates and haemorrhages

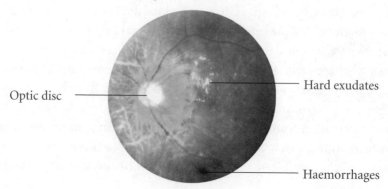

Optic disc

Hard exudates

Haemorrhages

It must be stressed that in diabetes not all blurring of vision is due to the abovementioned conditions. It can sometimes be due to fluctuating levels of blood glucose when the eyes have to constantly adjust to the fluctuating density of the lenses. This may make you think that you need to change your spectacles (if you are already wearing them), although that would be of no use. When you are not sure, it is wiser to seek medical advice, in case any of the conditions mentioned earlier is developing.

Other diabetes-related eye conditions include corneal abrasion, decreased corneal sensation, paralysis of eye muscles causing double vision, and optic nerve damage due to poor blood supply to the nerve.

REGULAR EYE EXAMINATIONS

The surest way to prevent diabetic eye diseases, apart from correcting the risk factors mentioned earlier, is to have regular eye checks. Eye checks are now commonly done using a retinal camera or by examination with an ophthalmoscope through dilated pupils (direct ophthalmoscopy). Caution: If you have glaucoma, dilating the pupil can further raise the eye pressure. Mention your glaucoma to your doctor.

Type 1 diabetics should have a retina examination within 3 to 5 years after diagnosis, whilst Type 2 diabetics should have it done at the time of diagnosis. It should then be repeated yearly (if no abnormality is detected) or earlier as decided by the doctor, or if you develop symptoms. With modern treatment, blindness due to diabetic eye diseases can be prevented if eye problems are detected early and treated appropriately.

TREATMENT

The cataract operation is a day-surgery procedure whereby the opaque lens is removed and replaced with an artificial one. The treatment of glaucoma is by medication, eye drops and/or surgery.

Timely laser photocoagulation and surgery is effective in arresting the progression of retinopathy. The objective is to destroy areas that are deprived of blood supply to prevent further sprouting of new vessels and, hence, prevent retinal and vitreous haemorrhage. The risk of making the vision worse is very minimal. Some deterioration in night vision and narrowing of the field of vision may result, but compared with the long-term benefit, this is a small price to pay.

When vitreous haemorrhage and retinal detachment occur, surgery is more intricate and difficult and has to be done under general anaesthesia. The haemorrhage is removed and the vitreous body replaced with a sterile fluid, a procedure called vitrectomy, while the detached retina is delicately put back in place. The success rate for restoring vision is, understandably, not as high as for laser surgery for a less severe stage of the condition.

Case 20: Mr BT – Don't Go 'Blur'

The light was unbearable as Mr BT stepped outside his doctor's office. Three years ago, he had had a reddish film of blood in his right eye and his doctor had informed him then that he had advanced retinopathy and needed immediate laser treatment. He recovered from that surgery. This time, the doctor noticed some blood in his left eye and informed him that the problem was worse. Mr BT had lived a life of uncontrolled diabetes, was smoking heavily, and it was very likely that he would develop this complication again. As he went for the surgery, he was very fearful of going blind and was relieved when his treatment was successful once again. Mr BT realised how close he had come to losing his sight. He resolved to control his diabetes, quit smoking and have regular eye checkups.

09 FOOT PROBLEMS AND FOOT CARE

"We are what we repeatedly do.
Excellence, then, is not an act but a habit."

—Aristotle (384–322 BCE)
Greek philosopher, scientist and politician

Diabetes is the major cause of non-trauma related leg amputations. This is because the diabetic person is at risk of getting foot ulcers, infections and gangrene (death of tissue from lack of blood supply, usually accompanied by infection). When antibiotics fail to arrest the infection, the limb often has to be sacrificed to save life. Hence, it is very important for the diabetic to look after his or her feet. The advice has oft been cited, "Look after your feet as well as you look after your face."

WHY DIABETICS ARE MORE PRONE TO GETTING FOOT PROBLEMS

This boils down to two chronic diabetic complications—peripheral neuropathy (damaging nerves in the legs and feet) and peripheral vascular disease (causing poor blood supply) related to long-drawn disease, chronically high blood sugar levels, smoking, high blood pressure and unfavourable lipid profile.

Peripheral Neuropathy

This develops insidiously. Symptoms are numbness, tingling and pain in the legs, feet and toes, followed by gradual loss of sensation. You then risk injuring your feet through friction with ill-fitting footwear or common daily injuries without realising it until it is too late.

Peripheral Vascular Disease (PVD)

This occurs in the context of generalised atherosclerosis, a condition in which the arteries are narrowed by cholesterol plaques. The early symptoms are aches and pains in the legs and feet. The site of the pain depends on the level of obstruction to blood flow. Initially the pain occurs during walking but, as the disease progresses, there is pain even when at rest. In extreme cases, PVD can lead to gangrene, in which the affected skin and underlying tissues, deprived of oxygen and nutrients, gradually become non-viable, turning black and setting the stage for infection.

EVALUATION OF DIABETIC FOOT PROBLEM

A typical examination of your legs and feet by your doctor or podiatrist includes testing them for sensation (to light touch, sharp pain, pressure, vibration and temperature), looking for abrasions, presence of calluses and corns (indicating areas of increased pressure), injuries, ulcers and deformities, and testing the strength of muscles and muscle reflexes. Blood flow to the feet and toes will be assessed by finger palpation or special bedside instruments. The health of the nails will also be assessed. Your shoes will also be examined for their suitability according to your foot shape and type, and presenting structural problem, if any. Special tests may be done to obtain details, e.g. doppler ultrasound scanning of the major arteries in your legs to find out the extent and severity of the blockage, and nerve conduction velocity tests to obtain details of nerve function.

TREATMENT

Although there are drugs that relieve the pain of peripheral neuropathy and peripheral vascular disease, treatment to restore nerve function is, at best, of limited effectiveness. Aspirin and other drugs that reduce blood clotting are useful in improving blood flow. In selected cases, blood vessels bypass or stenting surgery, much like for coronary arteries blockage, can be done to restore blood flow, relieve pain and improve wound healing. Treatment of foot ulcers rests on appropriate wound care and the selective use of antibiotics and the use of pressure relieving insoles/shoes.

PREVENTION OF FOOT PROBLEMS

Prevention is of paramount importance and cannot be overemphasised. This is what you can do:

- Maintain good control of blood glucose, lipids and blood pressure.
- Do not smoke.
- Seek early treatment for foot problems.
- Take care of your feet.

Taking Care of Your Feet

- Keep your feet, toes, and the spaces in between your toes clean by washing with lukewarm water and using mild soap.
- Dry your feet by patting them gently with a soft towel, not forgetting the spaces in between the toes, as dampness predisposes to abrasion and fungal infection.
- Use a gentle moisturising cream for dry skin, but avoid the space between the toes. As moisturisers on the soles may make them slippery, applying moisturisers before going to bed is safer.
- Apply baby powder, if your feet tend to sweat excessively.
- Trim your toe nails properly. Trim nails straight across and not by following the curves of the edges, to avoid developing ingrown toe nails. Trimming the nails is easier after a bath as they are softer. Get someone else to trim your nails if you have poor eyesight, to avoid injury. As an alternative to nail clippers or scissors, you can also use a nail file to trim the nails.
- Inspect your feet and toes daily, looking for cuts, scratches, skin abrasions, corns, blisters, sores, ingrown toenails, discoloration and any changes in skin temperature.
- Consult your diabetes care team, especially your podiatrist, if foot lesions do not heal within a reasonable time, or when you are in doubt of their significance.

Self-treating Mild Injuries or Wounds

- Clean the injured area well with an antiseptic solution or sterile sodium chloride 0.9% solution. (Do not use Dettol because it contains alcohol and may injure the surrounding healthy tissues.)

- Cover the clean wound with a sterile dressing. Make sure the edges are stuck down properly so that no bacteria can get in to infect the wound.
- Check the wound every day. If it is not getting better within 2–3 days, or you notice redness, swelling, pus, throbbing pain or have a fever, get medical help from your doctor or podiatrist immediately.
- Keep pressure off the site of a wound or ulcer.

What Not to Do
- Do not use mercurochrome, iodine or traditional remedies for wounds (as the colour change may hide any infection or inflammation).
- Do not use strong chemicals or antiseptics, such as hydrogen peroxide.
- Do not use corn plasters.
- Do not prick or burst a blister (keeping the overlying skin intact protects it from infection).
- Do not apply heating pads or dip your feet in hot water or use a hairdryer to dry your feet.

Footwear
Never go barefoot outside or even at home if you have decreased sensation in your feet. Here are some simple rules on footwear:
- In general, wear clean, firm, covered shoes whenever practical. Sandals or slippers may expose your feet to injuries. Sport shoes or special 'diabetes shoes' are ideal if you have peripheral neuropathy. Proper fit cannot be overemphasised. As a general rule, there should be a space of 2 cm (one thumb width) between the longest toe and the front interior of the shoe. If your feet are of unequal length get the shoe size that fits the longer foot. Check for signs of improper fit, such as redness caused by friction, especially when wearing new shoes. All new footwear should be given a break-in period and not worn for long periods straight away. Do not use a new pair of footwear for any holiday trip.

- Socks should, preferably, be cotton to promote the absorption of moisture or of synthetic fibre to wick away moisture if you have sweaty feet. Do not wear socks or stockings with tight elastic bands. Change your socks daily to reduce the risk of infection.
- Check the insides of shoes and socks, before wearing them, for any objects that may injure your feet, especially if your sensation to pain is not very good.

LEG AND FOOT EXERCISE

Walking improves blood flow to the legs and feet. This should be a daily routine for all people, but for the diabetic with early symptoms of peripheral vascular disease, it is even more important as it can improve blood circulation and prevent worsening of the condition. Swimming, cycling and static rotation and upward and downward bending of the ankle will also help.

FINAL FOOTNOTE

The main focus should be on prevention. Dr Elliot P Joslin, founder of the world-famous Joslin Diabetes Centre in Boston, once said, "I am convinced that diabetic foot ulcers are not heaven-sent but Earth-borne." There is, indeed, much that you can do to preserve the health of your feet and legs.

10 FASTING AND DIABETES

"Life is a sum of all your choices."

—*Albert Camus (1913–1960), French novelist,
essayist, playwright and philosopher, Nobel Laureate*

DAWN-TO-DUSK FASTING

People with diabetes may want to undergo periods of fasting for religious reasons, such as Muslims during the month of Ramadan. This chapter pertains specifically to the dawn-to-dusk fasting observed by Muslims.

Limited studies have shown that severe hypoglycaemia is more common when Muslim diabetics observe this optional fasting. At the other end of the spectrum, the risk of hyperglycaemia and diabetic ketoacidosis in Type 1 diabetes is also higher because of a tendency to overeat and to reduce physical activity and medications from a fear of hypoglycaemia. Weight changes are variable, ranging from weight loss or no change to weight gain at the end of the fasting period. Dehydration is also a potential threat.

Guidelines[1]

Experts have put forward management guidelines for dawn-to-dusk fasting and caution those wanting to undertake it that they should be aware of its risks. You should always seek the advice of your diabetes care team before embarking on a fasting programme.

Do Not Fast if You Fall under the Following Circumstances:

- Type 1 diabetes
- Recurrent hypoglycaemia or severe hypoglycaemia within the last 3 months

- Hypoglycaemia unawareness
- Recurrent diabetic ketoacidosis or hyperglycaemia hyperosmolar syndrome, or such an episode in the past 3 months
- Poorly controlled or unstable blood sugar
- Severe diabetic complications, such as heart disease, kidney failure and kidney stones
- Severe hypertension
- Ongoing infection
- Pregnancy or breast-feeding
- Elderly, frail, and on insulin, especially if you are living alone.

Fasting is Relatively Safe if:
- You do not fit into any of the abovementioned situations
- Your diabetes is being treated by diet alone or by medications that do not stimulate insulin secretion
- Your weight is within or above your ideal weight range
- Your blood sugar levels are stable
- You are prepared to closely monitor your blood sugar.

Although the rules are quite strict, it is a common observation that many Muslim diabetics choose to go through with the fasting, despite not fulfilling the above safety guidelines.

FASTING AND DIET
Follow a proper diet plan given by your dietitian. During the fasting hours, your liver still makes sugar to keep you going. So, you do not need to eat extra when you break fast. Also, fasting should not be an excuse to take sweet foods and drinks, such as dates, cakes, biscuits and sugared soft drinks during the 'feasting' period. Here are some rules to observe:
- Drink enough fluids to prevent dehydration (if not during the fast, then before the fasting period).
- Sugars (such as glucose tablets, regular soft drinks, candies, chocolates, table sugar, etc.) should only be taken during hypoglycaemia (Refer to Chapter 6).

- If you cannot resist taking simple carbohydrates (like those mentioned above), it is better to take them in the sunset meal.

FASTING AND EXERCISE

In general, light exercise is safe if you are not on insulin but avoid strenuous activities. Always have with you some sugar source to treat hypoglycaemia when necessary. The best time to exercise is 1 to 2 hours after the evening meal. It can also be done after the morning meal but, as lunch will be skipped, there is a higher risk of hypoglycaemia in the afternoon, as the effect of exercise on the blood sugar can be quite prolonged. Exercising just before sunset is not advisable because you will be more prone to hypoglycaemia at that time of the day. The dosages of insulin and other diabetes medications will have to be reduced.

FASTING AND DIABETES MEDICATIONS

During fasting, some medications may not be suitable and your doctor might have to make changes to the type, dose and timing of your medications.

Oral Diabetes Tablets[1]
Refer to Chapter 3, Part 4.

Drugs that Stimulate Insulin Secretion
These include tolbutamide, glibenclamide, glipizide, gliclazide, glimepiride, repaglinide, and nateglinide.

If you normally take any of these medications once a day (e.g. glimepiride) the dose may have to be reduced.

If you normally take any of these medications twice a day (e.g. glibenclamide, glipizide, gliclazide) and the evening dose is less than the morning dose, the dosage should be reversed.

If it is normally taken three times a day (e.g. tolbutamide, repaglinide, nateglinide) and, because you now have to compress the three doses into two, you may have to combine the morning and mid-day doses and take it at sunset when you break the fast and take the usual sunset dose in the morning before you start your fasting, or simply skip the mid-day dosing. Long-acting sulphonylureas, such as chlorpropamide (seldom used now), should not be used during fasting.

Drugs that Do Not Stimulate Insulin Secretion

These drugs include metformin, rosiglitazone and piogligtazone. They are less likely to cause hypoglycaemia. For metformin, which is normally taken twice or thrice a day, the dosing should not exceed twice daily. You may then have to combine the mid-day with the evening dose. Total daily dose is best split into one-third in the morning and two-thirds at sunset.

Drugs that Reduce Intestinal Absorption of Carbohydrates

Acarbose can still be taken with each meal during the 'feasting' time (with breakfast and dinner).

Incretin Enhancers or DPP-4 Inhibitors

These include sitagliptin and vildagliptin. They are less likely to cause hypoglycaemia and the dose need not be changed although no studies have been done for dawn-to-dusk fasting.

Insulin[1]

Insulin treatment is a potential cause of hypoglycaemia during fasting. Appropriate modification of timing and dosage is usually necessary. In general, less insulin is needed during the day since lunch is skipped.

Four regimens can be used (with caution):
1. Regular short-acting insulin or rapid-acting insulin before breakfast and dinner and intermediate-acting insulin at bedtime.
2. Regular short-acting insulin or rapid-acting insulin before breakfast and intermediate plus regular short-acting insulin or rapid-acting insulin before dinner.
3. Long-acting (Glargine or Detemir) with regular short-acting insulin or rapid acting insulin before breakfast and dinner.
4. Premixed insulin (e.g. Mixtard 30HM, Humulin 30/70, NovoMix) before breakfast and before dinner. Most of the time,

the diabetic observing dawn-to-dusk fasting and already on this regimen will simply reverse the usual regimen, that is, the usual higher morning dose is used when breaking fast at sunset while the smaller evening dose is used in the morning.

These regimens, however, do not guarantee smooth blood sugar levels throughout the day. Discuss with your doctor which regimen best suits you. This is because during the fasting hours, the liver will continue to make glucose and if the body does not have enough insulin, the blood sugar level can still be quite high. On the other hand, if the morning insulin includes an intermediate insulin (as in any of the premixed insulin mentioned above), hypoglycaemia in the afternoon may occur.

It is, therefore, necessary to monitor your blood sugar frequently and to make adjustments accordingly. For example,

- If hypoglycaemia occurs in the afternoon, your intermediate-acting insulin dose at breakfast (which peaks 4 to 12 hours after injection) should be reduced.
- If hypoglycaemia occurs a few hours after your breakfast, your regular short-acting or rapid-acting insulin taken before sunrise should be reduced.

WHEN TO BREAK THE FAST

Terminate the fast when:
- Hypoglycaemia occurs (blood glucose less than 3.3 mmol/L)[1].
- Your blood glucose is less than 3.9 mmol/L in the first few hours after the start of the fast, especially if insulin, sulfonylurea drugs, or meglitinides are taken at predawn[1].

BLOOD SUGAR MONITORING

- When fasting, test your blood sugar levels regularly (at least 2 to 3 times a day);
- When you break fast, test your blood sugar level 2 to 3 hours after eating.

CHECKING FOR URINE KETONES

As blood sugar may remain high despite fasting, checking for ketones is necessary to detect impending diabetic ketoacidosis (DKA). Check for the presence of urine ketones when your blood sugar is above 16 mmol/L.

MONITORING BODY WEIGHT

Make sure you do not gain or lose weight too quickly during this period.

AFTER THE FASTING PERIOD

- See your doctor with your record of blood glucose levels.
- Take note of any changes in your diabetes treatment.
- See your dietitian for a review of your meal plan.
- Continue monitoring your blood glucose levels at home as you gradually return to your normal lifestyle.

To conclude, when you have learnt how to balance your meals, oral medicines, insulin and activity levels, and are prepared to observe the safety rules, you can go ahead with dawn-to-dusk fasting. Do remember that the potential complications are real. Therefore, you must put in greater effort to make the necessary adjustments.

11 SEXUAL HEALTH

"When we are no longer able to change a situation,
we are challenged to change ourselves."

*—Viktor Frankl (1905–1997), Austrian-Jewish neurologist,
psychiatrist, psychotherapist and Holocaust survivor*

Sexual problems related to diabetes are more common than they are openly discussed. Diabetes is no different from any illness in causing a damper on your libido, sexuality and sexual potency as a result of anxiety, fear, stress and depression, and these can, of course, be aggravated by other general factors, such as work stress, financial difficulties and relationship problems.

Sexual problems due to purely psychological factors can be overcome as you come to terms and learn to cope with diabetes. On the other hand, such problems can also be a manifestation of nerve and blood vessel damage.

If you suspect that your sex life has been affected by diabetes, discuss the problem with your doctor.

ERECTILE DYSFUNCTION IN MEN

Although, in men, infection of the penis, or balanitis, is not uncommon when blood sugar is not well controlled and personal hygiene not observed, the main issue often centres around sexual impotence or erectile dysfunction (ED) which is characterised by difficulty in getting and maintaining an erection. It is estimated that 50% of diabetic men have ED. Non-psychological or organic ED can be differentiated from psychological ED by its gradual, rather than sudden, onset and by the absence of nocturnal or early morning erection. It usually occurs 10–15 years after the onset of diabetes.

Causes of Diabetes-related Erectile Dysfunction (ED)

Psychological Factors
Anxiety, fear, depression, work stress, financial difficulties and relationship problems.

Blood Vessel Damage
The healthy penis becomes rigid by being filled up with blood during sexual arousal. Poorly controlled diabetes causes ED because of damaged and blocked blood vessels in the penis.

Nerve Damage
Penile erection is normally controlled by specific nerves. These nerves need to function normally to transmit arousal signals to the brain, which then send signals down to the blood vessels of the penis to increase blood flow. Long-standing, poorly controlled diabetes damages these nerves. This is one of the manifestations of the generalised diabetic peripheral neuropathy mentioned in Chapter 2.

Although in diabetics the disease may be the primary cause of ED, several other factors contribute to and aggravate the problem. These are:

Cigarette Smoking
Cigarette smoking accelerates the process of damage to the blood vessels, including those of the penis. It is another reason to stop smoking.

Alcohol Consumption
The belief that a drink or two improves sexual prowess and performance is not true. Chronic and heavy exposure to alcohol damages the peripheral nerves, much as chronic, poorly controlled diabetes does. This is called alcoholic peripheral neuropathy. This may also be aggravated by certain vitamin deficiencies frequently encountered in those who drink regularly and heavily. Like smoking, this is yet another reason to stop or restrict alcohol consumption if you have diabetes.

Medications

People with diabetes are often being treated for associated high blood pressure. Some of these antihypertensive drugs may impair erection. Sometimes, the problem can be traced to a particular medication, in which case the solution is simply to stop the medication or switch to an alternative, if it does not compromise your blood pressure control. Check with your doctor if you suspect that your high blood pressure pills are affecting your sex life. However, do not just stop these medications on your own, as this action may be harmful.

Hormone Disorders

Impotence may, sometimes, be unrelated to your diabetes. It may be due to other hormonal disorders, such as thyroid disease, high prolactin levels and sex hormone deficiency. If there is any clinical suspicion, your doctor might check the levels of these hormones in the diagnostic work-up. These hormonal conditions are managed differently.

Available Treatments for Erectile Dysfunction

Doctors do not routinely inquire into your sexual health. Therefore, it is up to you to open the discussion, if it is important to you. Your doctor may suggest a particular treatment or refer you to a specialist.

The introduction of drugs called PDE5 inhibitors (PDE refers to phosphodiesterase, pronounced: 'fos-fo-dai-es-te-race') has revolutionised and simplified the treatment of male impotence in diabetics and non-diabetics. These drugs increase the calibre of the blood vessels by increasing levels of nitric oxide in the penis. Available in the market are sildenafil (Viagra®), vardenafil (Levitra®) and tadalafil (Cialis®). They may cause headache, nausea, vomiting and visual disturbances (flashes of light and bluish tinged vision). They can also cause serious heart problems, especially when taken with nitrates, such as glyceryl trinitrate, isosorbide dinitrate and isosorbide mononitrate.

The PDE5 inhibitors have largely replaced more invasive and costly treatments, although some of these are still available from urologists and some endocrinologists. Such treatments may be considered when the PDE5 inhibitors are not effective or contraindicated. These more invasive treatments include self-penile injection of prostaglandin, vacuum pump devices (which create a negative pressure around the penis to draw in blood into the penis), and penile implant which can be filled up with saline via an implanted reservoir to give it rigidity.

WOMEN'S ISSUES

- In women, more so than in men, associated obesity, seen in Type 2 diabetes, can lead to a low self-esteem of the woman's physical image and sexuality.
- A decline in libido due to purely psychological factors, such as anxiety, fear, depression and stress, is generally similar to that affecting the diabetic man, although the woman will have issues specific only to her gender.
- Poorly controlled diabetes may cause irregular menses.
- Women with diabetes also need to deal with the effects of changes in appetite and sex hormones on blood sugar levels at different phases of the menstrual cycle. During the week before the menstrual period, blood sugar can be higher than usual because of food craving or hormonal influence during the second half of the cycle.
- Diabetes can result in more frequent vaginal yeast infection and urinary tract infection, particularly when blood glucose control is poor.
- Peripheral neuropathy, when present, reduces sensitivity of the skin around the vagina area and thus reduces arousal and pleasure.
- Vaginal dryness can make sexual intercourse unpleasant and even painful. Many factors contribute to this problem: poor diabetes control, reduced blood flow to the vagina due to generalised atherosclerosis, and menopause.
- Oral contraceptive pills contain either oestrogen plus progestogen or only progestogen. They can adversely affect blood sugar and lipids.
- Pregnancy and childbearing is more demanding and stressful for the diabetic woman, compared to the non-diabetic, as the anxiety of having a less than healthy baby hangs over her

all the time. (More on pregnancy and diabetes in the next chapter.)

- Menopause and the months leading to it can cause mood changes and hot flushes with sweating. These symptoms may be confused with hypoglycaemia and lead you to eat more than you need, thus affecting diabetes control.
- Note that hormone replacement therapy (HRT) during menopause, contrary to previous belief, has been shown, in recent years, to increase the risk of heart attack and breast cancer. Therefore, its use to alleviate menopause symptoms has to be weighed carefully.

What You Can Do

- When low libido and impaired sexual arousal are due to purely psychological factors, the help of a clinical psychologist should be considered.
- Medicated lubricants are effective and simple remedies for vaginal dryness.
- Do frequent blood glucose tests and keep records of your menstrual pattern and any related symptoms and discuss them with your diabetes care team.
- You may need adjustments to your medications, including insulin, during periods that regularly cause your blood sugar to be high or low.
- Blood pressure and lipid levels should be watched more closely when you are on oral contraceptive pills.

SEXUAL ACTIVITY AND HYPOGLYCAEMIA

This issue, of course, affects both men and women. Sexual activity is, after all, a form of physical exercise. It does not usually cause your blood glucose to drop significantly. However, it is conceivable that in the well-controlled diabetic on medications, hypoglycaemia can occasionally occur.

The usual rules of prevention and treatment of hypoglycaemia in non-sexual physical activities apply (see Chapter 3 Part 3 and Chapter 6). It may not be the most romantic prelude to sex to do a blood glucose test or even to take a carbohydrate snack before or after sex. However, when necessary, such precautions may save you from some unpleasant experiences during and after what is intended to be a pleasurable and fulfilling activity.

IMPOTENCE – BEYOND SEX

As sexual problems, such as impotence, may be related to diabetic peripheral vascular disease and diabetic neuropathy, the diabetic person who suffers from them will do well to pay equal attention to other areas that may be simultaneously affected by poor blood flow and nerve damage, such as the heart and feet.

12 PREGNANCY AND CHILD-BEARING

"You give but little when you give your possessions.
It is when you give of yourself that you truly give."

—Kahlil Gibran (1883–1931), Lebanese-American poet,
writer, artist, sculptor and painter

Let's begin on a positive note. It is now possible for a woman with diabetes to have a healthy baby, thanks to improvements in diabetes management, monitoring of the unborn child and neonatal care (the first four weeks after birth).

However, it is still important to realise that diabetes does make the pregnancy more difficult and that there is a higher risk of miscarriages and birth defects. Babies born to diabetic women tend to be larger than average (macrosomia), posing delivery problems. Macrosomia is due to excessive production of insulin by the unborn child in response to the high sugar it gets from its mother, as insulin promotes growth. These babies are also more prone to develop neonatal hypoglycaemia, again due to the excessive insulin which takes a few hours to be cleared away after the child is delivered. There is also a greater risk of the baby developing neonatal jaundice and breathing difficulties, due to immaturity of the liver and lungs respectively, especially if the baby has to be delivered before term. These potential problems can be reduced with planning and meticulous care of your diabetes.

PLANNING FOR A BABY

The decision to have a baby when you have diabetes has to be made carefully and in consultation with your doctor. If you already have any of the chronic diabetic complications mentioned in Chapter 2, these complications do sometimes get worse during pregnancy. For example, pre-existing diabetic retinopathy needs to be stabilised before pregnancy, as it may worsen during pregnancy. Ironically, this is sometimes due to improved diabetes control with more intensive insulin treatment. Likewise, an already weak heart may be further overburdened by pregnancy. Severe diabetic kidney disease may also worsen high blood pressure and predispose to pre-eclampsia. The good news is that any worsening of diabetic complications, if they occur, usually reverts to the previous stage after the pregnancy, unless the damage has resulted in permanent functional loss, such as severe retinal haemorrhage.

After you have weighed the risks and decided to go ahead with having a child, it is very important that you get good control of your blood sugar before you conceive. This means a HbA1c as near as possible to that of a non-diabetic person, or less than 7%[1]. Inform your doctor or your diabetes care team about your plans.

If your diabetes control is still poor, some form of contraception is advisable until it gets better. Studies have shown that good preconception control of diabetes results in fewer birth defects than if you start controlling your blood sugar only after pregnancy is known. A HbA1c of more than 1% above normal in the first 6 to 8 weeks of pregnancy results in more birth defects than you expect to see in the general population.

MEDICATIONS

The safety of all oral anti-diabetes medications has not been fully established, although glyburide (or glibenclamide) and metformin are relatively safe in studies done so far. Nonetheless, it is still recommended that Type 2 diabetic women on oral medications be transitioned to insulin as soon as a decision is made to conceive, and certainly as soon as pregnancy is confirmed.

Insulin is still the safest option during pregnancy. Intermediate-acting isophane or NPH insulin, regular short-acting insulin and rapid acting insulin analogues, such as insulin lispro and insulin aspart, can be used. However, because the safety of the long-acting insulin analogues, glargine and detemir, is still not established, these latter two insulins have to be transitioned to NPH insulin.

Other medications, such as the ACE-inhibitors and ARBs (see Glossary) for blood pressure control and kidney protection, and statins for lowering cholesterol, should be stopped prior to conception and throughout pregnancy as they may cause foetal defects and complications.

With good planning, you will have a better chance of having a healthy and safe pregnancy.

TYPES OF DIABETES IN PREGNANCY
Pre-gestational Diabetes
First of all, the word 'gestation' refers to the period of the foetus's development from fertilisation to birth. The term 'pre-gestational diabetes' is used when a woman had diabetes before getting pregnant. Therefore, one could have either 'pre-gestational Type 1 diabetes' (or 'Type 1 diabetes in gestation') or 'pre-gestational Type 2 diabetes' (or 'Type 2 diabetes in gestation'). If you have the latter and now need insulin, it does not change the fact that you are still a Type 2 diabetic.

Gestational Diabetes Mellitus (GDM)
Some women did not have diabetes (or had not been diagnosed with diabetes) until they became pregnant. They are, then, said to have gestational diabetes mellitus (GDM). True GDM does not have the chronic complications of diabetes.

GDM occurs because the pancreas is not able to produce enough insulin to overcome the insulin resistance that occurs in pregnancy, as a result of the insulin-opposing hormones produced by the placenta. It usually occurs between the 24th and 28th week of pregnancy. It is more common in women who are overweight, above 35 years of age, have a family history of diabetes, or had large babies (4 kg and above) in a previous pregnancy.

If you have any of these risk factors, your obstetrician will check your blood glucose as soon as you become pregnant and, if it is normal, it will be checked again between the 24th and 28th week of pregnancy. If the test results are borderline, an oral glucose tolerance test (OGTT) will be carried out. The diagnosis is, then, based on the fasting blood glucose and/or blood glucose two hours after taking a 75 g glucose drink.

Based on the WHO criteria, GDM is diagnosed when the fasting blood glucose is 7.0 mmol/L and above and the 2 hours blood glucose 7.8 mmol/L or above. (The American Diabetes Association recently recommended slightly different blood glucose criteria, using the 100-g OGTT or 75-g OGTT, for the diagnosis of GDM.)

If you have GDM, your blood sugar usually normalises after the child is born, but there is a higher chance of diabetes developing in future with subsequent pregnancies (that is, a second GDM) or even in the absence of pregnancy. In some women, the diabetes persists after pregnancy. An oral glucose tolerance test (OGTT) is routinely done 6–12 weeks after the child is born, to determine this.

TREATMENT

More so than in other situations, you will have to work very closely with your doctors (diabetologist and obstetrician), diabetes nurse educators and the dietitian to achieve the best control with a minimum risk of hypoglycaemia.

For Pre-gestational Diabetes
Type 1 Diabetes

If you are a Type 1 diabetic, during the first three months, you may be more prone to low blood sugar. After that, the blood sugar tends to be higher than before pregnancy, especially during the last three months of pregnancy, as hormonal changes diminish the actions of insulin. Expect an increase in your insulin doses for blood sugar control. The most appropriate insulin regimen for you may be one that consists of four injections daily (see Chapter 3 part 5). Insulin requirement drops dramatically during labour and after the child is born.

Type 2 Diabetes

Mild cases, previously on diet control, can sometimes be continued on the same strategy. If control is not satisfactory, you will be put on insulin if the blood glucose levels are above recommended values (fasting blood glucose above 5.2 mmol/L, one-hour post-meal blood glucose above 7.2–7.8 mmol/L and two-hour post-meal blood glucose above 6.6 mmo/L). If your diabetes has been controlled with anti-diabetes tablets, your doctor will switch the treatment to insulin injections. The insulin regimen is variable and you may require up to four insulin injections daily.

For Gestational Diabetes Mellitus (GDM)

When diet and exercise fail to maintain adequate control (see above), you will need insulin. In general, the insulin regimen is usually less complex than for pre-gestational diabetes.

Some women with GDM over-diet in order to avoid insulin. This is not advisable, as it will cause your body to burn more fat and proteins to provide energy. The excessive burning of fats produces high levels of ketones in the blood, which may be harmful to the developing child.

EXERCISE DURING PREGNANCY

Yes, you may exercise during pregnancy, although this may sound surprising to some. The rules on exercise in Chapter 3 Part 3 are generally applicable, such as consulting your health care team prior to starting an exercise programme, pre-exercise warming up and post-exercise cooling down, checking blood glucose, avoiding dehydration, etc.

Exercise in moderation. Pregnancy is not the time to start an exercise that is too strenuous or that you are not accustomed to. Avoid activities that require holding your breath, jerky movements, body twists, and straining. Brisk walking, jogging, stationary bicycling, swimming and water aerobics are suitable. As your body's centre of gravity has shifted during pregnancy, there is a risk of losing your balance, so be careful to avoid falls.

BLOOD GLUCOSE TARGETS IN PREGNANCY

The blood glucose targets are more stringent in pregnancy than in non-pregnancy states (see Table 16). You need to work closely with your diabetes team and obstetrician to achieve the best possible control.

There is no short cut and the only way to achieve consistently good control is frequent self-blood glucose checks, up to seven times a day (three before-meal and three after-meal tests plus one at bedtime and/or 3 am), a few days a week.

Table 16: Blood glucose targets during pregnancy[2]

Timing	Ideal blood glucose* (mmol/L)
Overnight, before meals, at bedtime	3.3–5.5
Peak post-meal (1–2 hours after start of meal)	5.5–7.2

*Blood glucose here refers to whole blood glucose. Self-monitored blood glucose is glucose measured in whole blood (as opposed to plasma).

These more stringent targets are to maximise the health of the child. It may, however, lead to more episodes of hypoglycaemia to the expectant mother. A question that is often asked is whether maternal hypoglycaemia is harmful to the developing foetus. The short answer is "no". The foetus is able to cope with it remarkably well, thanks to the efficiency of the placenta to ensure that it gets enough glucose. Nonetheless, the mother should do her utmost to avoid hypoglycaemia without compromising too much on the blood glucose targets. It is, indeed, like walking a tight rope.

GOOD PRINCIPLES AND PRACTICES

1. Follow the recommended diet. Take frequent but small meals, that is, breakfast, mid-morning snack, lunch, mid-afternoon snack, dinner, mid-evening snack and bedtime snack. This way, the blood sugar will not fluctuate too much.
2. Regular exercise, if permitted.
3. If you are on insulin, take it as prescribed by your doctor.
4. Test your blood sugar levels 5 to 7 times daily, several days a week. If your diabetes has stabilised, less frequent testing may be alright, but only as advised by your doctor.
5. Work closely with your doctor or diabetes care team with regards to all the above issues.

ALCOHOL, DRUGS AND OTHER MEDICATIONS

You should stop smoking and drinking alcohol before you conceive and throughout the pregnancy. Smoking and alcohol can seriously harm your baby. Many medications can also be harmful to your baby. Check with your diabetes care team before taking any prescription or over-the-counter medications.

AFTER DELIVERY

GDM usually goes away after the child is born. If you had required insulin during the pregnancy, insulin can usually be weaned off very quickly.

If you have pre-gestational Type 2 diabetes, whether you can return immediately to your oral diabetes pills depends on whether you are breastfeeding or not, as not all of your usual pills have been shown to be safe for your breastfeeding child. You may have to continue on insulin for a while. If you have pre-gestational Type 1 diabetes, your blood sugar levels may have wide fluctuations. It may take a few weeks before they stabilise.

Although you will now have to cope with your newborn, you should not neglect your diabetes but ensure that you remain well for your own and your child's sake. Continue to check your blood sugar a few times a day. Maintain a healthy balance between your food and diabetes medications. Ensure that your food intake is adequate to prevent hypoglycaemia and yet not excessive as to undo the effect of diabetes medications. Exercise should resume as soon as you are physically up to it.

Your Baby

The chances of having a healthy baby are better if you have had good control of your diabetes before conception and throughout the pregnancy. If, on the other hand, control has not been good, the immediate postnatal care may be more protracted, if any of the complications mentioned at the beginning of this chapter is encountered.

Whether you have pre-existing diabetes or GDM, the risk of your child getting diabetes in later life is slightly higher (since he may have inherited your diabetic genes) but this is not invariable, as it also depends on trigger environmental factors. There is also evidence that babies with higher than normal birth weight born to women with GDM are more prone to becoming overweight in later childhood, especially if their parents are overweight. These children should, therefore, be encouraged to eat healthily and exercise regularly to prevent diabetes.

Breastfeeding

Breastfeeding is good and we encourage it. Breastfed babies of women with GDM, especially if the latter are overweight, are less likely to grow up overweight. The implication is that breast milk appears to counter the 'influence of the mother's obese genes'.

Breastfeeding, however, may be a nutritional drain on you. Your food is now shared with your baby, therefore be alert to potential hypoglycaemia. You will have to take more carbohydrates, apart from other nutrients such as proteins, calcium, iron and vitamins. You should also try to time your meals and snacks about half to one hour before you breastfeed. Watch out for cracked nipples and breast infections, as infection is always more of a risk in diabetics than in non-diabetics. If in doubt about your nutritional needs, speak with your dietitian.

Short-term small studies have shown that oral diabetes pills, such as glyburide (or glibenclamide) and metformin are safe during breastfeeding, as very little of the drugs end up in the milk. There is no similar data with regards to the thiazolidinediones. However, as *long term* safety has not been clearly established, oral diabetes medications are not recommended during breastfeeding.

Postnatal Visits

Do not miss postnatal visits to your doctor. If you had GDM, an oral glucose tolerance test (OGTT) is necessary 6–12 weeks after delivery to find out if the diabetes has gone or is persisting. About 15% of women with GDM continue to have raised blood glucose after pregnancy.

FUTURE RISK OF DIABETES MELLITUS

Studies have shown that women with GDM have a 30–70% risk of getting GDM again in subsequent pregnancies and about 10–15% risk of developing Type 2 diabetes within five years. Hence, annual screening for diabetes is recommended.

Case 21: Mdm SV – Get a Healthy Baby

Mdm SV burst into tears when her doctor told her that her baby was unusually large at 28 weeks of her pregnancy. She could not believe that she had developed gestational diabetes. Mdm SV had a strong family history of diabetes but always thought that she would never get it. She was devastated. The dietitian started her on a meal plan but her blood sugar levels were still very high. Subsequently, she was put on insulin and learned how to do blood sugar monitoring at home. Determined to achieve good control and to avoid complications, she learnt how to adjust her insulin dose according to her blood sugar results. Her efforts paid off and she successfully delivered a healthy 3.2 kg baby.

CONTINUING YOUR BEST EFFORTS

The demands on the pregnant woman with diabetes are definitely greater during pregnancy—more frequent visits to her health care providers, more blood glucose testing, keeping to a meal plan and exercise. However, the rewards of a smooth pregnancy and a healthy child are well worth it.

My observation is that pregnancy is a period when a woman takes the utmost care to control her diabetes (with few exceptions) because she knows it is in the best interest of her child. Relatively less effort on the part of the diabetes care team is needed to get her to follow the management plan. This speaks volumes of a woman's mother-instinct.

If your diabetes journey has taken you through pregnancy, you are likely to have learnt and discovered many aspects of diabetes management that you might not have known before, such as the finer points of matching your diet to the insulin schedule to maintain normal blood sugar. These are useful lessons that you should continue to put into action throughout the rest of your diabetes life (and not wait till the next pregnancy).

13 TRAVELLING WITH DIABETES

> "If one does not know [to] which port one is sailing,
> no wind is favourable."
>
> —*Lucius Annaneus Seneca (c4BC–AD65)*
> *ancient Roman Stoic philosopher, statesman and dramatist*

People with diabetes can travel and enjoy holidays or go on business trips like everyone else. It only takes some planning and preparation to ensure a safe and pleasant trip.

PLANNING IN ADVANCE

Before a long trip, visit your doctor, ideally 4–6 weeks before departure, to assess and optimise control. Bring along your itinerary, indicating departure and arrival time, duration of flights and time differences between points of embarkation and disembarkation. This will help your doctor advise you on the timing and dosing of insulin, if necessary. Obtain an official note from your doctor stating your diabetes status, what medications (including insulin) you are on, and what glucose meter you are carrying with you. This will spare you a lot of unexpected hassle at the immigration checkpoint. Inform the airline of special meal options and find out the times when in-flight meals are served.

MEDICINES AND DIABETES SUPPLIES

- Work out the quantity of medicines, syringes, insulin needles, test strips and finger-prick lancets you will need. Pack an extra week's supply in case of loss or a delayed return. Keep a list of all the medicines and diabetes accessories that you are currently using.

- Bring along your blood glucose meter with an extra battery and your record book.
- Pack some simple carbohydrate sources (such as glucose tablets and candy) for treatment of hypoglycaemia and some complex carbohydrate sources (such as snack bars) in case of meal delays.
- Pack your medicines and accessories in your carry-on hand luggage. This is to avoid being caught without all these essentials should checked-in baggage go missing. Moreover, extremes in temperature in the cargo compartment may spoil your insulin.
- Do not keep insulin in the glove compartment or in the boot of your car if the vehicle is left under extremes of environmental temperatures. In places where temperatures or humidity are very high, use special thermal insulated insulin travel packs to keep the insulin cool.
- Bring a doctor's prescription for your medicines, in case you need to replenish them.

DIABETES IDENTIFICATION
Wear or carry some identification to state that you have diabetes. This will enable other people to know how to assist you in times of emergencies such as hypoglycaemia.

CUSTOMS CLEARANCE
Bring a letter from your doctor stating your diabetes status and your medications and diabetes accessories. Certain countries (e.g. USA) may require that passengers also bring the original insulin box or packaging that displays label and pharmacy instructions. It is safe for your insulin or insulin containers to go through the X-ray machine. If in doubt, request for a manual check of your bag.

VACCINATIONS
If you need to be vaccinated for your overseas trip, do so well in advance. This is because you may feel a little unwell after immunisation and controlling your diabetes under this situation will be easier at home than during the trip.

TRAVELLING COMPANIONS

- If you are travelling with others, inform them about your diabetes. They should learn how to recognise hypoglycaemia and how to treat it. Ensure easy access to your diabetes identification.
- If you are travelling alone, let the crew or tour guide know about your condition.
- You might want to bring along this book, *The Diabetes Companion*!

MORE GENERAL TIPS

- Monitor blood glucose every 4 to 6 hours while in flight.
- Keep yourself well hydrated with non-alcoholic, caffeine-free drinks.
- While in flight, you do not have to inject air into the insulin bottle when drawing insulin. This is because the pressure in the cabin is usually lower than at sea level. By injecting air into it, the pressure in the insulin bottle becomes relatively higher compared to the cabin pressure, thus making it harder to control the plunger when you are drawing out the insulin, and more than the desired amount of insulin may be drawn into the syringe.
- Learn how to say, "I have diabetes" in the language of your destination. It may make a difference between life and death.
- Know well the place you are visiting, especially the locations of medical facilities and pharmacies.

MEALS ON BOARD AND ADJUSTING INSULIN DOSES

Inform the airline that you have diabetes a few days before the flight. You can request a special meal that is low in sugar, fat or cholesterol. A letter from your doctor or dietitian will help. With some airlines, you can even make your request online.

Trips that Cross More Than Five Time Zones

For long journeys, remember that when flying west, you gain time, the day is longer and more insulin may be required. On the other hand, when flying east, you lose time, the day is shorter and less insulin is required.

Apart from time zone differences, specific adjustments are also dependent on time of departure, flight duration and your current insulin regimen.

Find out the times when meals are served. Keep the time on your watch according to the point of embarkation till you arrive at your destination. Ideally, you should take your meals and snacks on board at the usual times, as if you were not travelling. The airline will usually be able to accommodate your request for meals to be served according to your needs if you inform them ahead. Check your blood sugar 4–6 hourly. Discuss with your doctor specific adjustments to your dosing schedule.

The following two cases will help to illustrate the above:

Case 22: Mdm RRN – Going to New Zealand with Diabetes

Mdm RRN was leaving Singapore at 8 pm for New Zealand, arriving at 3 pm NZ local time (10 am Singapore time). She was on Humulin N® (40 units pre-breakfast and 44 units pre-dinner) and NovoRapid® insulin (12–16 units before each meal). She was also on metformin (thrice a day taken after meals). She requested advice on how to manage her diabetes and insulin treatment on board.

- She should plan ahead so that she can finish checking in by 6.30 pm and have a leisurely dinner at the airport. She should give herself the usual evening insulin at the usual doses, assuming no major change in her dinner.
- While in flight, she should keep to Singapore time.
- She should not take the first in-flight meal which is likely to be served between 10 pm and 11 pm (as it is not her usual meal time).
- At the usual breakfast time, say 8 am Singapore time, she should ask for her breakfast. Her Humulin N® should be halved (that is, 20 units), as it would by then be 1 pm in NZ. Her NovoRapid® insulin dose should be as usual (less if the meal is lighter). After arrival in NZ, at dinner time (local time) she should have the other half of the Humulin N® (20 units). Her pre-dinner NovoRapid® insulin dose can remain unchanged.
- The following day, she should resume the usual insulin schedule.

Other Tips:
- If she wants to take a meal or snack outside of normal times, extra NovoRapid® may be required.
- Her metformin schedule need not be changed.
- Blood glucose levels should be checked every 4 to 6 hours during the flight.

Case 23: Mr JN - Going to London with Diabetes

Mr JN, a well-controlled Type 1 diabetic, was travelling to London from Singapore, leaving at 11.20 pm and arriving at 5.50 am London time (almost 2.00 pm Singapore time). He was on Insulatard® (20 units before breakfast and 16 units before dinner) and Actrapid® (8 units before breakfast and 8 units before dinner).

- On the evening of his departure, his dinner Insulatard® and Actrapid® insulin should be taken as usual.
- He should keep to Singapore time throughout the flight.
- As a full meal is served between 1 and 2 am (5 and 6 pm in London), he should give himself a small dose of Actrapid® (4–6 units) if he would like to take it. However, it is better that he resists taking it, as it is not usual for him to take a full meal at that time.
- If it is his norm to have a bedtime snack to prevent nocturnal hypoglycaemia, he should just take a snack and not the full meal.
- At breakfast time (8 am Singapore time, midnight in London), he should ask for his breakfast. He should then give himself half his usual morning Insulatard® (10 units)—since it would be midnight in London—plus the usual 8 units of Actrapid®.
- At the next meal time, at 4 am London time (noon, Singapore time), it is best that he skips the meal. If he would like to have it, he should take the meal with 4 units of Actrapid® only (half the usual dose).
- After arrival, it is recommended that he begins his insulin schedule according to London time, around 8 am, with his usual 20 units of Insulatard® (as his last Insulatard® was 12 hours earlier) and 8 units of Actrapid® followed by his breakfast. (If he has eaten the 4 am breakfast with Actrapid®, he should take 4 units of it for this meal.)

The above two scenarios are just examples. The exact insulin dose adjustments have to be individualised.

Trips that Cross Fewer Than 5 Time Zones:

There is, generally, no need to adjust your insulin dose during these shorter trips.

Eastward Journey

After your arrival, because your day has been 'shortened', eat a little extra carbohydrate after your next insulin injection, as there may be some lingering insulin from the last injection.

Westward Journey

One approach is to make no changes to your insulin before departure, but because the day is longer, the insulin you have taken may not last up to your arrival when you begin your new time schedule. Check your blood glucose and if it is high, take an extra dose of regular short-acting or rapid-acting insulin.

TRAVELLING WITH ORAL MEDICATIONS

In general, the timing of oral diabetes medications is not as crucial as for insulin. Dose adjustment will depend on the types of medications used.

If you are on only metformin, acarbose or rosiglitazone (either on its own or in combination with one another), you can continue taking them at the usual dose and time (based on embarkation point) while in-flight without any worry of hypoglycaemia. Acarbose has, of course, to be taken with meals and not apart from them.

If you are on twice or thrice daily sulphonylureas (e.g. tolbutamide, glibenclamide, glipizide, gliclazide) and travelling east, it might be safer to skip the in-flight dose instead of taking the medicines too close together (because of the timing of the in-flight meals) and risk getting hypoglycaemia. When flying west, skipping a dose may cause slight hyperglycaemia.

If you wish to keep to twice daily sulphonylurea medications, when going across more than five time zones, take half the usual dose on board at the usual time (based on embarkation point) and the other half after you have arrived, based on destination time.

With regards to medications such as repaglinide and nateglinide (that act like sulphonylureas but are taken on per meal basis), they can be taken as usual on board, as long as that is followed by a main meal.

* * *

Bon voyage! Have a great and normoglycaemic holiday!

14 COPING WITH DIABETES AND YOUR EMOTIONS

*"Living fearlessly is not the same thing as never being afraid.
It's good to be afraid occasionally. What's not good is living
in fear, allowing fear to define who you are.
Living fearlessly means standing up to fear, taking its measure,
refusing to let it shape and define your life."*

—Michael G Ignatieff (1947–)
Canadian award-winning writer, professor and politician

DEALING WITH YOUR EMOTIONS

At the beginning of this book, we alluded to the reality that, for many people, the diagnosis of diabetes is like the sky falling down on them. Shock, denial, anger, rebellion, fear, anxiety and depression are common initial reactions that can lead to treatment neglect. These are what we would call 'diabetogenic emotions,' that is, emotions that make you lose control of your diabetes. (For an inspiring story, refer to the case of Mdm YLF in the Introduction.) You have to learn how to deal with these powerful diabetogenic emotions that surface from time to time.

Adjusting to the demands of diabetes is a continual process. There are suddenly so many changes to make. You have to watch your diet, start exercising, watch your weight, take pills or injections, monitor your blood sugar, and visit your doctor. Every moment of your day seems to be centred around diabetes. It is with you all the time, twenty-four hours a day, seven days a week, and it does not look like it is going away. Just about anything related to your diabetes keeps playing in your mind: stigma, blindness, sexual impotence, early death, hypoglycaemia, financial drain, losing job, rejection by friends, the whole gamut of 'life's unfairness.'

Do you feel overwhelmed by the constant demands of caring for your diabetes? Do you worry constantly about your blood sugar, but still feel unmotivated to do something about it? Do your moods go up and down like your blood sugars? Do you feel like giving up?

If you feel like this, you are not coping very well. No matter how long you have had diabetes, bring it up with your diabetes care team, instead of keeping it to yourself.

Signs of coping well:
- Eating right and having enough sleep
- Daily physical activity
- Fulfilling work and hobby
- Positive and hopeful

Signs that help is needed:
- Over-eating
- Over-drinking
- Withdrawing from others
- Negative thinking
- Depression

Fear and Anxiety

Ignorance, they say, is bliss but it can be dangerous. However, on the other hand, as you learn more about diabetes and become more aware of its complications, you might become fearful and anxious. Whilst a small dose of fear can sometimes be a good motivator, driving you to achieve good control, too much fear can also be paralysing. See the section below on developing a positive attitude.

Frustration

Sometimes, you feel like you are on a roller coaster. For a few weeks, you manage to go on a strict diet and exercise routine. Then, one night, you slip up and reach out for that chocolate; one piece leads to two, and then to three. So, not only does your blood sugar go on a roller coaster spin, your emotions do too, as you feel guilty, angry, frustrated and depressed. You lose your motivation and think: "What's the use of trying?" and feel like giving up.

Diabetes Burnout

You can get burned-out from the seemingly endless rounds of tests, visits to the doctor, estimating calories, watching your weight and remembering to take your pills. It gets worse when your doctor, nurse or dietitian insinuates that you are not doing your best. (Don't be upset; take a step back and make a list of the things that you are doing that are helpful and not helpful. Then choose one or two small things to change.)

Ironically, you can also get burnout when you are too strict on yourself and are going for perfection. Strike a healthy balance and set small, achievable goals.

DEPRESSION AFFECTS DIABETES

Are you depressed? Do a self check using the table below:

Table 17: Depression checklist

Warning signs of depression		
Persistent low or sad mood	Yes	No
Loss of interest or pleasure in daily activities	Yes	No
Feeling tired all the time, lack of energy, poor concentration	Yes	No
Lack of drive or motivation that makes even simple tasks difficult	Yes	No
Agitation, restlessness, irritability	Yes	No
Sleeping too much or too little	Yes	No
Withdrawing from friends or social activities	Yes	No
Feeling useless, inadequate, helpless or hopeless	Yes	No
Frequent thoughts of suicide or death	Yes	No

If all or most of your answers to this checklist are 'Yes', you could be depressed. When you are depressed, it is difficult to take good care of yourself and do all the things you're supposed to do. Depression adversely affects your diabetes control by upsetting the good routine of self-care activities, diligently learnt from your diabetes care team. Some of the symptoms of depression, such as lethargy, poor concentration and low moods may be confused with fluctuating blood sugar. It is a vicious circle that must be broken as soon as possible. If you feel depressed and cannot cope, talk to your diabetes care team. You may need the help of a mental health professional, as in the case of Mdm FBA.

"Life is not a matter of having good cards, but of playing a poor hand well." This quote by Robert Louis Stevenson reminds us that we should learn to play the game to the best of our abilities despite the odds. But be careful not to become so compulsive that your life is focused only on diabetes. Take a break now and then. Believe that you can have a good and fulfilling life nonetheless.

To think positively, you have to look out for the negative thoughts and change them to positive and encouraging ones. For example, challenge your negative thoughts by asking yourself:

- Have I jumped to conclusions?
- Am I being too hard on myself?
- Am I too much of a perfectionist and being unrealistic?
- Am I blowing things out of proportion?
- Is there another way to see this situation?
- What would I tell a friend if he/she were in the same situation?

Table 18: Negative and positive ways of looking at a situation

Situation	Negative thoughts	Positive thoughts
When you have a setback	I have failed, I'm useless. Why even bother to control my diabetes?	Just because I slipped up does not mean that I am a failure. What can I learn from this setback? Are there better ways to meet my goals?
When you feel overwhelmed	It is all too much. I can't handle it.	Let me take it one step at a time. What is the first thing I need to do?
When you feel guilty	I should not have eaten that *char kway teow*, I am so useless, I can never stick to my diet.	Am I shouldering too much blame? What did I manage to do that was OK?
When you feel ashamed	If people know I have diabetes, they will pity me and think I'm abnormal.	I am not the only one with diabetes. Maybe I can ask around and see who else has it.

JOIN A SUPPORT GROUP

No matter how long you have had diabetes, do not deal with it alone. Living with diabetes is a lifelong journey. Support and help from other people can make the stress much easier to handle.

Share your feelings or worries with your family, friends, or diabetes care team. Talk to other people who have diabetes too. You might be surprised to find out how many people have diabetes and are living well! Join a diabetes support group to get tips on how to cope with diabetes. However, do bear in mind that another person's state of diabetes may be different from yours—different routines and different medicines that may not always apply to you. Refer to the 'Resources' chapter for a list of local support groups.

Case 25: Ms MT – Others Have Overcome, So Can You!

Ms MT had Type 2 diabetes and her control had been deteriorating gradually. Her doctor started her on oral diabetes tablets and had been sending her for many rounds of diabetes education. She just could not see the need for diabetes education. She kept saying, "I'm not silly! I know all this stuff! What a sheer waste of my time!" The diabetes team was convinced that she was denying the seriousness of her diabetes but was still very patient with her. They allowed her to ventilate and express her thoughts and feelings about diabetes.

Then, she read an article in the newspaper. She found that her favourite actress had diabetes for years and once went into a coma for a week because of very high sugar levels. However, through proper diet control, regular exercise and insulin treatment, this actress was able to control her diabetes. By taking better care of herself, she was able to live her life fully. The story struck a deep chord in her and MT realised that she was not helping herself with a negative attitude. She finally came to terms with her condition and promised not to ignore her diabetes before it was too late.

TAKE FIVE—LEARN TO RELAX

"Every now and then, go away, have a little relaxation,
for when you come back to your work,
your judgement will be surer."

—*Leonardo da Vinci*

Too much worry and stress can upset your blood sugar levels because the hormones your body produces in response to stress oppose the actions of insulin and are, therefore, diabetogenic (remember this word at the beginning of this chapter?).

Have a balanced lifestyle and do things to feel good:
- Take short breaks.
- Take up a hobby.
- Do relaxation exercises (see the box below).

- Schedule enjoyable activities in your life.
- Chat with friends at your favourite coffee shop.
- Spend more time with people you like (do these include your health care providers?).

Relaxing the mind and body

Try this simple relaxation technique to unwind and de-stress. Set the mood by taking your time. Do not rush to relax. You should take a shower first, if you are home. Put on comfortable clothes. Choose a quiet place. Play soft music you enjoy.

Once the mood is set, practise calm breathing:
1. Take in a normal breath through your nose with your mouth closed.
2. Exhale slowly.
3. When exhaling, say the word 'RELAX' very slowly, as in: "R-E-E-E-E-L-A-A-A-A-X-X."
4. Count slowly up to four, then inhale again, and repeat the steps above.
5. While breathing slowly, imagine a place of beauty and serenity that you enjoy. It can be a beach, a forest, a mountain, anything you fancy. Try to picture it as vividly as possible—the details, the smell, the sounds, your feelings, and enjoy it.
6. Do this exercise several times a day, taking 10–15 breaths at each practice.

Practise, practise, practise—relaxation is a skill which needs to be learnt.

BOUNCING BACK IN 10 STEPS

Take the following steps every time stubborn diabetogenic emotions rear their ugly heads:

1. Recognise

Recognise that negative emotions are natural and normal. Tell yourself that the totally carefree diabetic is a myth. Everyone with diabetes struggles with it.

2. Share

Share your feelings with your diabetes care team, family, colleagues or friends.

3. Accept

When you accept your diabetes, you learn to take control of it instead of letting it control you. You can handle the frustrations and failures better. Think of your 'different' or 'complex' lifestyle as a healthy lifestyle that is good for everyone. Yes, you might even be able to influence your non-diabetic family members and friends to adopt your healthy lifestyle.

4. Move on

Move on as soon as you have aired your feelings.

5. Learn or re-learn

Perhaps there are some things that still puzzle you. Perhaps you are not injecting your insulin correctly. Go back to the relevant sections of this book. Share with your diabetes care team all the questions and worries that are on your mind. Other people with diabetes can also teach you a thing or two but always remember that their situation is never exactly the same as yours.

6. Identify the problem

If you are having difficulties controlling your diabetes or feeling overwhelmed, ask yourself: "What is the issue?, What is the hardest part for me right now about controlling diabetes? Is it diet, testing my blood sugar or exercise?" Denying a problem does not make it go away.

Be specific. For example: "I keep forgetting to check my blood sugar every morning." Or "When I'm stressed, I just can't resist snacking on butter cookies."

7. Find solutions

Use your past experiences to help you find a solution to a current problem. Was there a time when your diabetes control was better? What did you do differently then? Has your diet changed? Were you taking your diabetes pills more regularly then? Should you do more blood sugar checks after a meal?

Your health care provider can help you find solutions if you share openly and honestly about your difficulties. It is alright to inform your diabetes nurse, instead of your doctor, if you feel more comfortable with her. She is often the best person to identify your fears and domestic and work problems. She is trained for that very purpose and will work closely with your doctor to try to find a solution.

8. Set realistic goals and "Just do it!"

By setting small, realistic goals, you are less likely to be disappointed. If it suits you better, focus on one goal at a time.

For example, do not aim to start an exercise programme by jogging one hour every day. Start with 15 minutes of brisk walking thrice a week and gradually increase the intensity and duration. You are more likely to achieve your goals if you make gradual changes.

The same goes for self-blood glucose monitoring. Over-ambition and aiming for perfection might cause burn-out. Once you have hit a realistic solution, stick to it, like Mr R in Case 26.

9. Reward yourself for your efforts

Give yourself a pat on the back whenever you achieve a goal, even if your doctor, nurse or dietitian forgets to congratulate you, in their busyness. If you have shed 1 kg in a month instead of the 2 you aimed for, give yourself credit for trying. Maybe you didn't manage to start exercising but you have switched from oily chicken rice to chicken macaroni soup and started eating more vegetables. Praise yourself for sticking to your meal plan! Give yourself a treat for making progress—a new pair of sports shoes, a movie, a new dress or even two seeds of durian! Just two, OK?!

10. Share again
This time, share your success formula with someone else!

Do you feel better now?

Case 26: Mr R – Find a Solution (Walk the Dog and Control the Sugar)

Mr R knew that his problem was that after dinner every evening, he would snack non-stop in front of the TV—nuts, bananas, chocolate, juice. He realised that one way to stop this habit was to find something absorbing to do after dinner. He decided to take over one of his domestic maid's duties—walking the dog after dinner every evening. He, thus, not only put in some exercise but also cut down his snacking to only once or twice a week and felt happier and healthier for it. The next thing he planned to do was to take the plunge and ask his wife to keep any extra food in the house out of sight.

15 HANDLING THE CHILD WITH DIABETES

"We cannot all do great things. But we can do small things
with great love. And together we can do something wonderful."

—Mother Teresa (1910–1997)
Albanian missionary and humanitarian, Nobel Laureate

Diabetes in children is mostly Type 1 diabetes. However, Type 2 diabetes in children and adolescents is becoming more prevalent because of increasing obesity as a result of growing affluence, overeating and more time spent in front of the television and computer.

This chapter will not be dealing with the nitty-gritty of diabetes management, as that is done by the paediatric endocrinologist/diabetologist. Instead, it will discuss what the family, especially the parents, can do to help the child and ease him/her into adulthood.

FACING REALITY

You may initially feel depressed, worried, guilty or even angry when your child or adolescent is diagnosed with diabetes. However, it is important for you to overcome your initial reactions to focus on how best you can help and support your child.

Be prepared that it will demand a lot of your time and energy. Educate yourself about diabetes and work closely with your child's diabetes care team. For example, you will need to spend time talking with your child's paediatrician, diabetes nurse educator, dietitian and other health professionals.

You might get stressed and will need the support of your spouse and other family members.

You may need to make changes to your work routine so that you can devote more time to your child.

To prevent yourself from burning out, remember to ensure that your own health and relationships needs are being met. Take breaks and do things you enjoy.

ENSURING A NORMAL CHILDHOOD

Children with diabetes are no different from other children in their physical, psychological, social, and intellectual development needs. Ensure that they are not neglected in any of these other areas.

If your child is very young, you will need to be more involved in his diabetes care routine. As soon as he is able to understand, teach him the basics of healthy nutrition, exercise, insulin injections and blood sugar tests.

Focus on what your child can still do, despite having diabetes, instead of what he cannot do.

Encourage him to engage in sports, outdoor and social activities, camps, holidays, etc., whilst also taking appropriate precautions and not neglecting his treatment routine.

Stay calm and positive so that he will also grow to have a positive attitude about his diabetes. While it is necessary to teach him about the complications of poorly controlled diabetes, try not to be overly anxious. Focus on the things he can do to gain control over his diabetes.

Your own confidence will promote confidence in your diabetic child. Do not be overly worried or protective or allow him to be too dependent on you. You can care for him and discipline him as with your other children without diabetes.

It is also important to encourage your child to share his experiences and feelings about living with diabetes, and for you to take time to listen, so that you can better understand and support his struggles and needs.

KEEPING DIABETES UNDER CONTROL

Most children with diabetes have Type 1 diabetes. In many ways, keeping blood glucose under control in children is not very different from that in adults.

Some basic rules:
- Have good meal planning—Children and their families must learn what types of food and drinks to avoid. Stock up on healthy snacks at home, instead of soft drinks and sweet juices.
- Check blood sugar levels regularly—Teach your child to use a blood glucose meter and keep a diary to record blood sugar levels.
- Regular exercise—Physical activity helps to lower blood sugar levels and helps children to control their weight. Teach them to check their blood sugar levels before starting a game/sport to prevent hypoglycaemia.

HYPOGLYCAEMIA

Repeated and severe hypoglycaemia in children younger than 5 years old may cause permanent cognitive impairment. Children younger than 7 years are more likely to have a degree of hypoglycaemia unawareness (see Chapter 6). Therefore, blood glucose goals for young children should be less stringent than those for adults (see Table 19).

Preventing and Managing Hypoglycaemia
- Children should take their meals on time and have appropriate snacks in between meals. They should be given something to eat when they show warning signs of low blood sugar, such as temper tantrums, sweating and shivering.
- Parents should stay calm and avoid over-reacting when their child gets hypoglycaemia. Having an emergency plan and educating yourself about what to do in such a situation can help you stay in control.

Table 19: Blood glucose goals for young children[1]

Age	HbA1c target	Pre-meal plasma blood glucose (mmol/L)	Post-meal plasma blood glucose (mmol/L)
Toddlers (up to 6 years old)	7.6–8.5%	5–10	5.5–11
6–12 years old	<8%	4.5–10	5–10
13–19 years old	<7.5%	4.5–7.5	4.5–8

IN SCHOOL

Inform your child's school about his diabetes, what treatment he is on and how the school staff can help. They should be aware of:

- Your child's need to take meals and snacks on time, even during class.
- The signs and symptoms of hypoglycaemia and how to manage it.
- The child's specific needs before undergoing physical or sports activities.
- Not discriminating your child on account of his diabetes.

GROWING UP

When your diabetic child grows into his teens, he will, naturally, be more self-conscious of his diabetes. He might feel embarrassed and think that he is different from his friends because of diabetes. He could also fear that friends may look down or laugh at him. He may become angry about his diabetes and act out or be more rebellious. He is likely to become more exposed to, and want to try, new experiences, such as smoking, alcohol, and sex. Peer acceptance is important. He is more sensitive about what his friends think of him, and friends may have more influence on him than family.

This is a period of change and turbulence, and you will have to be patient and understanding. Diabetes care means following strict routines and most teenagers have problems coping. This can cause teenagers to become frustrated with, or to ignore, their diabetes. Parents will need to balance between wanting to supervise and control the teenager's actions and inculcating in him a sense of responsibility versus allowing him to be more independent.

Be alert to signs of eating problems (either binge eating or extreme dieting) in your child/teenager. She (usually girls) may skip insulin to avoid putting on weight (as insulin does have this side-effect). Focus on developing a positive relationship with your teenager, so that he will be open to your guidance. Show interest in his activities and hobbies, and listen without being judgmental.

Case 27: LM – Teenager with Diabetes (I)

Mdm Tan was worried about her 16-year-old daughter, LM, who had diabetes for five years which, until recently, had usually been well controlled. She seemed to have lost interest in her diabetes and had stopped doing her blood sugar tests. Her last HbA1c reading had shot up and the doctor thought she was missing some insulin injections.

Case 28: DT – Teenager with Diabetes (II)

Mr and Mrs Tong's 15-year-old son, DT, developed diabetes when he was ten. Initially, he was very sensible about his diabetes but, recently, he had become resentful, saying that he was different from all his friends and blaming his parents for his condition.

The situations of LM and DT are, unfortunately, not uncommon. Their parents could help by, amongst other things:

- Lending a listening ear, letting the teenager express his frustrations and difficulties.
- Encouraging and praising the teenager, for example, praising him for diabetes care tasks done, even if it is only the occasional checking of blood sugar. This will usually gradually improve his self-motivation.
- Not nagging, criticising or threatening the teenager when he does not stick to the diabetes care plan. Forcing strict compliance may cause him to hide things from you.
- Being tactful when bringing up the problems with the teenager's diabetes care team.

TRANSFER OF CARE

At this stage, your teenage child may still be under the care of the paediatrician or be transferred to an endocrinologist in adult medicine. His own preference should not be ignored, as he is more likely to be cooperative with regards to his treatment if he feels comfortable with his doctor.

When he is transferred to the adult health facility, after the initial few visits, unless it is necessary for you to be present, allow him to see the doctor on his own. Squabbles between the teenager and his parents and between parents over all sorts of diabetes issues are not uncommon during consultations. However, continue to be involved and supportive in his treatment in a non-intrusive way.

16 INTERACTING WITH YOUR HEALTH CARE PROVIDERS

"Coming together is a beginning. Staying together is progress. Working together is success."

—Henry Ford (1863–1947)
American industrialist and founder of the Ford Motor Company

THE TEAM

The management of diabetes is increasingly complex, and you are likely to have interacted or will be interacting with more than a few health care professionals, as well as other people with diabetes. Your primary physician may be the neighbourhood or company general practitioner (GP), a doctor in a neighbourhood government polyclinic, an Internal Medicine specialist, a diabetologist, a general endocrinologist, or even a cardiologist.

How many and whom you have to interact with depends on many things, such as the state of your diabetes control, your predominant problem and your preferences. In the Singapore context, your diabetologist, if you need one, is an endocrinologist (a specialist in the field of disorders of hormones and hormone-secreting glands). He or she, in all probability, treats not only diabetes but also many other disorders of hormones, such as thyroid diseases.

Other health professionals helping you along the way will be the dietitian, the diabetes nurse educator, the general nurse, the podiatrist, the pharmacist, the clinical psychologist and a host of other specialists, depending on your needs.

A good working relationship with all of these professionals goes a long way towards a smoother walk with diabetes.

You Hold Centre Stage

One fact is inescapable—you are not only part of the team but also the main player in this multidisciplinary interaction. You and you alone decide how many slices of that yummy toast bread or how much of mum's *mee rebus* you should be eating; whether you will go for an evening brisk walk instead of watching others sweat it out on the Amazing Race; how often you want to test your blood sugar, whether you are going to see the GP about that blister on your heel, and so on.

Case 29: Mr KNK – "The Ball is In Your Court"

Forty-seven-year-old Mr KNK has had diabetes for 10 years and had been taking insulin for the last five years. His diabetes control was good, initially, with his HbA1c around 7%. However, for the past two years, his HbA1c had increased to anything between 8.6% to 14% because of a failure to fully comply with the insulin schedule. He and his wife were puzzled and concerned about his weight loss of 5 kg. He admitted that he would often skip his once-a-day long-acting bedtime insulin (glargine) whenever he had a late dinner when his pre-dinner short-acting insulin (aspart) would also be late. He feared that the bedtime glargine was too close to the pre-dinner aspart. (He was reassured and accepted that this should not be a concern.) He had also been routinely skipping his pre-lunch insulin aspart injection as it was "not convenient" to inject at his place of work.

At the end of the consultation, he conceded that, although work was hectic, he had enough time for lunch. And since he had his own office, he could administer his injection out of sight of his colleagues before he joined them for lunch. He knew that 'the ball was in his court' and heeded his doctor's advice about taking his insulin at lunchtime.

Distributing the Care: The Right Person for the Moment

While it is reasonable to expect the best from every member of your diabetes care team, remember that they are working within the constraints of their specific training and practice and the local health system.

You can also expect them to communicate with each other as needed. Many will readily admit that there are certain areas which they are not sure of and which they will need time and the assistance of colleagues to find a solution to your problem. It is in the interest of everyone that you go to the appropriate health care facility or health care provider for any particular problem.

Case 30: Ms GT – "Consult the GP? Sure, Why Not?"

Ms GT, whose diabetes was recently given a clean bill of health by her diabetes doctor, developed a painful red patch on her left little toe after a minor scratch. Frantically, she called our Diabetes Centre nurse to get an earlier appointment to see her diabetes specialist. As the doctor's list was quite full for the next two weeks, she was advised to see a GP in the meantime, and she did so, albeit reluctantly.

When she finally got to see her diabetes specialist, the pain had gone from the toe, which had only a residual pinkish colour. From the photo of the lesion, taken with her handphone camera, what she had was cellulitis (a superficial skin infection), which had responded to the antibiotic given by her GP. She was still very effusive, almost complaining, about how she should have been allowed to see her diabetes specialist at the Diabetes Centre straightaway, instead of going to the GP.

Her specialist was not to be flattered and took the opportunity to educate her that we gave her the right advice on the right course of action. In medicine, we call this the 'right siting' of health care.

Consultation with Your Specialist

While a holistic approach to your health needs is ideal, there is only so much time you have with your diabetes specialist. Maximise it to sort out any diabetes and diabetes related issues.

Scenario One

You have sprained your wrist and have a touch of food allergy, or so you think. Your scheduled appointment with your diabetes doctor is a week away. You have sought treatment from a GP whilst waiting to see your diabetes doctor. When you finally get to the diabetes check-up, use the consultation time wisely to focus on important issues. If the sprain and allergy are already responding, albeit not completely, to treatment by your GP, it is wiser to spend the time discussing your recent spate of hypoglycaemia than to dwell on the wrist and the allergy, which your diabetes doctor is not the best person to treat anyway!

He has noticed that your high HbA1c does not gel with the, mostly normal, blood sugar readings on your home monitoring chart that you faxed over recently. While the doctor would do well to be sympathetic about your sprained wrist and allergy, he and you will have to focus quickly on the diabetes issues within the short consultation time, so that a solution can be found. The cause of your reported hypoglycaemia needs to be diagnosed and treated and your glucometer and your testing techniques also need to be checked.

Scenario Two

If you have chronic insomnia, none of your diabetes care team members is likely to be more qualified than your neurologist to comment on whether you should go through a sleep study for chronic insomnia; therefore, asking them for a second opinion should be a low priority or not done at all.

YOUR INPUT

Getting your blood sugar, blood pressure and fats under control is a dynamic affair, to say the least. The three therapeutic pillars are diet, exercise and medications. Do not be offended if your doctor, nurse or dietitian probes into your adherence to these measures.

All therapeutic decisions/actions are taken based on your feedback on the relevant issues and the results of tests. Your diabetes care team members recognise that therapy burn-out is a reality and make allowances for that. But they need to know the truth to be able to make rational decisions to improve control. Making decisions based on false or incomplete feedback, such as increasing your diabetes medications, can be hazardous.

The doctor cannot assume that the medicines he last prescribed are exactly what you are currently taking. To assume so may be disastrous. If there has been any change (subtraction or addition), the onus is on you to mention it, even before he asks you. It is vitally important that your communication is clear. Know your medications absolutely. If drug names are beyond you, write them down on a piece of paper or bring along the medicine for quick and easy reference. Likewise, clear records of recent self-monitored blood glucose are very useful for a clear understanding of your condition.

Going to the consultation with clear and relevant information saves both parties not only a lot of time and exasperation but can also prevent therapeutic mishaps! (Refer to Case 13 in Chapter 5, where the patient falsified his blood glucose records.)

Towards a More Rewarding Consultation

Go prepared. Be clear about what specific health issues you have, so that the consultation will be worth it and done with the minimum of fuss. Your health care providers work within their specific training and the constraints of the local health care system and are not without their flaws. Nonetheless, two hands are always needed to clap.

Here are some commonly neglected issues and what you can do to help your health care provider serve you better.

Questions

If you have any questions for your doctor, nurse or dietitian, list them down if you are likely to forget them.

Self-monitored Blood Glucose

If you have been asked to do self-blood glucose monitoring (SBGM), try your best to do it and bring along the chart. If the readings are still in the glucometer, transfer them to the chart for easier analysis. Bring along the meter, in case your doctor or nurse needs to check that it is functioning properly and that you know how to use it.

Letters, Memos and Notes

Bring along any recent hospital discharge summary or any relevant notes that might have been passed to you by other doctors. These are important for the continuation of care.

Blood Test and Other Tests

If blood tests are scheduled, bring along the lab forms.

1. Fasting blood glucose

Fast overnight if you have been asked to do so. You will have to delay your diabetes medicine and/or insulin until the blood has been drawn. However, you should still take your other medications (with plain water) before leaving home, such as blood pressure tablets. Bring along your diabetes tablets and/or insulin. After the fasting blood test, have your breakfast and take the diabetes tablets and/or insulin accordingly.

2. Random (non-fasting) blood glucose

If a random blood glucose test has been ordered, take your meals and medications as usual before coming. Your doctor will sometimes want to know your random (non-fasting) blood sugar. He may want to know what it is after a meal, be it breakfast or lunch.

3. Timing of tests

In many health facilities, blood and urine tests results are available within 15 minutes to a few hours, depending on what is tested. There may be occasions when you need tests that take a few days to give the results. In such cases, you will be asked to come for the tests a few days or a week prior to your check-up.

Some patients mistakenly assume that all blood tests must be done after an overnight fast and before a meal. When their consultation is in the afternoon, they skip their breakfast and lunch (!) and all medications, including blood pressure tablets, resulting in a high blood pressure reading when they see their doctor.

Medications

Know your current medications, especially if you have any questions about them, or if there have been changes made since your last visit. Write them down if you have difficulty with the medical terms. Better still, bring them along with the labels (not as loose pills which may be almost impossible to identify). If you have excess medications that you do not want to waste, know the number of tablets/vials of insulin, so that it is easier for your doctor to work out the shortfall that you have to collect.

At the end of the consultation, pay careful attention to any changes that your doctor has made. Jot down the changes, if necessary, especially the insulin doses. The pharmacist will go through them with you once more when you collect the medicine. Refer to the instruction labels again when taking the medications.

Names and Dates

In this modern age of specialisation, you may be seeing more than a few doctors at various clinics. Know the names of these clinics, specialties, doctors, nurses as well as your next appointments with these various health facilities. This will assist your doctors and nurses to better coordinate your treatment.

THE RELATIONSHIP

If you feel that your health care provider is 'scolding' you, try to remember that he does not mean it, and that you would not want to have someone looking after your health to be impassive about your sugar, blood pressure or fat readings, or adopt a totally liberal and permissive attitude and merely hope for the best. The doctor who 'scolds' you is often, also, the one who will readily congratulate you when your health improves through your own efforts.

Then again, there are instances when patients thank their doctors for 'scolding' them into action when they realise that their own actions count more than anything else. Or a spouse asking the doctor to 'scold' the patient for being undisciplined in following the treatment plan.

At the end of the day, what really matters is your improved health. Nonetheless, like other human relationships, a particular doctor-patient relationship may not always be as comfortable as you would like it to be and the scope for moving on to a new relationship is always open to you. Doctors are enlightened enough to accept that and will not feel offended. They even believe that that may actually be for the mutual good! Remember, however, that doctors advise you and act in your best interests, so do not confuse pleasing words with good clinical outcome.

17 ALTERNATIVE MEDICINES AND SUPPLEMENTS

*"Destiny is not a matter of chance, it is a matter of choice.
It is not a thing to be awaited for, it is a thing to be achieved."*

—*William Jennings Bryan (1860–1925)*
American politician, orator and lawyer

In the pursuit of health, longevity and relief from ailments, people who are already taking 'conventional' Western medicines often seek alternative therapies, and those with diabetes are no exception. They are often attracted to various forms of health supplements, such as vitamins, or traditional therapies, such as Chinese herbal and Ayurvedic medicines, although many of these are not currently recommended because of the lack of proven efficacy[1].

It is estimated that, across cultures, 17–72% of people with diabetes use complementary and alternative medicine, and this could include herbal and nutritional supplements, spiritual healing and relaxation techniques.[2]

A survey[3] of 600 diabetic patients in 2000 at the Diabetes Centre of Singapore General Hospital revealed that 12% had used or were using herbal products for diabetes. About 80% of those surveyed did not inform their doctors about the usage, and one-third spent more than S$100 a month on these alternative medicines.

One major concern is that many would try these often ineffective alternatives or even replace their usual conventional diabetes treatment with these supplements.

This chapter is not to be viewed as a tacit encouragement to use these alternative therapies, but to give you general information on the subject. If you cannot resist taking or are currently taking alternative medicinal products, inform and discuss the subject with members of your diabetes care team, including your pharmacist. Check out the facts, separate myth from truth, and keep out of harm's way.

IS THE SUPPLEMENT SAFE?

In early 2008, a variety of mysterious pills made headlines in Singapore when they caused severe hypoglycaemia in men taking them for sexual enhancement[4]. These unlicensed products, purportedly made from natural sources, were very soon found to contain glibenclamide (an oral diabetes medication, see Chapter 3 Part 4) at doses several times that used for diabetes, and sildenafil (the active ingredient in Viagra, see Chapter 11). They went by different names, such as Power 1 Walnut and Power 1 Singapore. At the time of writing, more than twenty men had been hospitalised for adverse effects (primarily hypoglycaemia) and five lives had been lost from hypoglycaemic coma, pneumonia, brain oedema (fluid swelling) and fits.

This recent event is reminiscent of another one, several years back, in which another unlicensed product, Slim 10, taken for weight loss, caused severe liver failure in some consumers. These are indeed grim reminders of the danger of taking unlicensed products that make bogus claims. Remember that 'natural' does not mean 'safe' or 'effective'.

SAFETY REGULATION

In Singapore, the regulation and sale of supplements and alternative medications is under the purview of the Health Sciences Authority (HSA). The HSA strives to ensure that Chinese Proprietary Medicines (CPM) are safe, of good quality and are appropriately labelled before they are allowed to be sold.

However, unlike for Western medicines, the effectiveness of CPM in treating a medical condition is not reviewed. Nonetheless, a particular CPM must not contain any Western medicine, nor exceed the limits set for toxic heavy metals, such as arsenic, copper, lead and mercury, and must not be contaminated with micro-organisms that can cause infections. Importers must submit test results for every consignment of CPM imported; HSA does not test every batch of CPM itself.

Unlike CPM, other traditional medicines (e.g. traditional Malay and Indian medicines), homeopathic medicines and health supplements are currently not subjected to pre-marketing approval and licensing for their import, manufacture and sale in Singapore. The responsibility for the safety and quality of these medicines and supplements rests with the manufacturer, importer and seller. The requirements for their safety are similar to that for CPM products, except that no approval is required from HSA. Hence, there is less regulatory oversight with regards to their stated ingredients. It is, therefore, even more important that these supplements come from reputable sources.

The HSA mandates that all CPM, alternative medications and supplements cannot claim to treat any of the 19 diseases/conditions specified in the First Schedule of the Medicines Act. The list includes cancer, diabetes, hypertension and sexual dysfunction. Any product that claims to be useful for these conditions without regulatory approval should be approached with utmost care and a huge dose of scepticism.

GUIDE TO USING SUPPLEMENTS AND ALTERNATIVE MEDICATIONS:

1. Know the name, dosages and effects of the products you use.
2. Tell your healthcare provider about the products you take. Some of these supplements may affect your medical condition or the medicines that you are taking.
3. Do not combine these supplements with prescription medications without informing your healthcare provider. Some supplements can affect your blood sugar levels, and can cause severe hypoglycaemia. Others can lower the effectiveness of your diabetes medications via drug-drug interactions.
4. Do not stop taking your prescribed medications without informing your doctor. These supplements have not been proven to substitute for your usual medications.
5. Know what benefits to expect after taking the alternative medication. If it does not work, stop taking it, despite its claim.

6. Add only one new product each time to see how this particular supplement affects you.
7. Record the doses and adverse effects of the supplement you use. Also note their effects on your blood sugar level. Stop using them if you experience adverse effects. Contrary to common belief, herbal medicines and supplements are not 100% safe and can still cause serious adverse effects.
8. Take note of the total daily dosages of the ingredients if you are taking more than one product containing similar ingredients. For example, calcium may be found in supplements that are taken for bone or joint problems, or in those designed for post-menopausal women.
9. Follow the stated dosage recommendations — more does not mean better. Taking additional amounts can mean exposing yourself to more adverse effects without increasing benefits.
10. Do not use supplements if you are pregnant or breastfeeding, unless you have verified with a health care professional that it is safe to use.
11. Do not give supplements to young children.
12. Stop taking supplements before surgery and other medical procedures.

VITAMINS

Many people with diabetes are attracted to vitamin supplements, not least, due to media hype. While the underlying defects of diabetes and diabetic complications are, in part, related to high levels of oxygen free radicals as a result of hyperglycaemia, and antioxidant nutrients, such as vitamins, do mop up these harmful radicals[5], the evidence is still sketchy and contentious that taking supplementary vitamins (including vitamins C, E and beta-carotene) makes a lot of difference in reducing the risk of diabetes progression and diabetic complications[6].

Moreover, excessive intake of certain vitamins is not without harm[6]. Vitamin E can increase the risk of bleeding if taken in excess, and in combination with blood-thinning drugs, such as warfarin. Beta-carotene excess may increase the risk of lung cancer and haemorrhagic stroke in men who smoke. Excessive intake of vitamin A or retinol may worsen pre-existing kidney failure and cause birth defects when taken during pregnancy. Under certain circumstances, it may behave, ironically, like an oxidant to make the 'bad' LDL-cholesterol even more atherogenic (i.e. more likely to block arteries).

If you have a well-balanced daily diet that includes a wide variety of fruits and vegetables, keep your blood sugar close to target, and are clearly not vitamin-deficient, you do not require any routine vitamin supplementation. A case, however, could be made for taking vitamin C supplements if you suspect you are not taking enough of it in your diet and if your blood sugar has not been in good control, as chronic hyperglycaemia increases urinary loss of vitamin C.

Remember that vitamin supplements, if taken, should be done in the context of a balanced diet and with the right dosing. It should not replace your usual diabetes and lipid medications, and adverse interaction with other drugs should be avoided.

ALTERNATIVE HERBAL THERAPIES

Many present day medications did have their origin in plant sources. In fact, a commonly used diabetes medication, metformin, was derived from the flowering plant French lilac[7], which was a common traditional remedy for diabetes in medieval times. However, many steps have to be taken to produce a medication from a plant source; therefore, not all crude extracts from plants containing known medicinal substrates are necessarily effective.

One of the concerns[8] regarding the use of herbal or botanical products relates to their interaction with the conventional therapy, causing either enhanced or diminished effect of the latter. The strength of these products also varies considerably, depending on which part of the plant or tree they are obtained from and on their formulation as capsules, tablets, liquid extracts or other forms. Even the geographical conditions of the source of these plants may affect the quality of the active constituents of the plant product. There may be several active ingredients which are pharmacologically effective only if taken together. Therefore, extracts of these individual ingredients may not have the same effect as that of the whole plant.

The clinical evidence for herbal products used in diabetes has mostly been inconclusive, and sometimes contradictory. Many claims of effectiveness are based on animal studies, or anecdotal reports (e.g. recommendations from a few patients), and studies involving only small numbers of patients or over a short duration.

A Cochrane (http://www.cochrane.org) database review of Chinese herbal medicines for Type 2 diabetes looked at 66 randomised trials, involving 8,302 participants. The review found that some mixtures of herbal medicines lowered blood sugar with no severe adverse side effects. Unfortunately, most of the included trials studied small numbers of patients and were of poor quality, making the results less reliable[1].

The way ahead is to await the results of large, randomised, placebo-controlled clinical studies of some of these traditional medicines to evaluate their claims of benefit.

BRIEF DESCRIPTIONS OF SOME HERBS AND SUPPLEMENTS

Gymnema (Gymnema sylvestre)

This is also known as *gurmar* in Hindi, which means 'sugar destroyer'. It reduces one's ability to taste sweet things after chewing the leaves. There is a long history of several centuries of chewing Gymnema leaves to treat *madhu meha* (honey urine) in Ayurvedic medicine. A member of the milkweed family, it is a woody plant found in tropical forests of India and Africa.

The exact way by which it works is not fully known, but believed to be by increasing glucose uptake and utilisation and enhancing insulin release. Animal studies suggest that some residual pancreatic function is required for this herb to work.

The scientific evidence for Gymnema comes from two non-randomised controlled trials conducted by the same group of investigators. In one study[9] a group of Type 1 diabetics on insulin taking Gymnema capsules twice a day saw their HbA1c improve significantly from 12.8% to 9.5% and their average fasting blood glucose fall from 232 to 177 mg/dL after 6–8 months. A comparator group given a placebo saw no improvement in their diabetes control. Sixteen to 24 months after the start of the study those still taking the supplement were able to maintain or see a further improvement in their diabetes control, but the study did not report the level of statistical significance. There was also a drop in insulin requirement in those taking Gymnema, but again the significance of this observation was not evaluated.

In another study[10], Type 2 diabetes patients taking sulphonylurea diabetes medication together with Gymnema had a significant reduction of their HbA1c from 11.9% to 8.4% and average fasting blood glucose from 174 to 124 mg/dL after 18–20 months, whereas those given a placebo registered no improvement. Five patients were able to discontinue sulphonylurea treatment.

Gymnema did not cause any more side effects than placebo in these studies, although it can be expected to cause hypoglycaemia if it is haplessly combined with other diabetes medications. Although these initial studies were promising, larger controlled studies are needed for more definitive answers.

Chromium

Chromium is an essential trace mineral that is found naturally in small amounts in some foods, including meat, fish, animal fats, coffee, tea, whole grain bread and some spices. In health supplement products, it occurs as chromium picolinate, chromium chloride or chromium nicotinate, most commonly as chromium picolinate. The Recommended Daily Allowance (RDA) for chromium is 20–35 mcg/day. Some multivitamins may contain 25–100 mcg of chromium per tablet.

Chromium plays an important role in glucose and fat metabolism. It may enhance the action of insulin action by increasing the number of insulin receptors and their binding to insulin. Although chromium deficiency has been linked to impaired glucose tolerance, most diabetics are not found to be chromium deficient.

So far, meta-analysis of studies on chromium supplementation did not show any concrete evidence of benefit except for the few done in China, in which chromium did improve blood glucose and HbA1c[11.]

In low doses, short-term chromium supplementation appears to be safe. Some patients may experience headaches, insomnia, sleep disturbances, and mood changes. Chronic use at high doses may be linked to blood disorders, liver problems and kidney failure.

According to the US Food and Drug Administration (US FDA), it is likely to be safe at a dose of 200 mcg/day for up to six months. However, there is insufficient safety data on its long-term use. There is also no easy and accurate way to measure chromium levels in the body to ensure the optimum dose.

Chromium may improve diabetic control, but should not be taken for more than six months or in high doses. It is probably not necessary as a supplement if you have a healthy, well-balanced diet.

Ginseng (Panax ginseng and Panax quinquefolius L.)

There are three different kinds of ginseng: Korean ginseng (Panax ginseng), American ginseng (Panax quinquefolius L.) and Russian/ Siberian ginseng (Eleutherococcus senticosus). Korean ginseng and American ginseng are the main ones studied for diabetes. Most often, the root will be used. The main pharmacologically active substance in ginseng are the ginsenosides. Historically, Korean ginseng has been used in TCM for a long time to treat diabetes

The exact mechanism of its action is unknown, but postulated to include slowing down of carbohydrate absorption, increasing glucose uptake by cells and increasing insulin secretion.

A study in 1995 on a small group of Type 2 diabetic patients suggested that ginseng may decrease fasting blood glucose and HbA1c[12]. A subsequent meta-analysis in 1999 concluded that the evidence for ginseng's health benefits was far from obvious[13]. More recent reports of its benefit for diabetes are small scale and sketchy.

Ginseng can cause nervousness and insomnia. Less commonly, irregular heart beats, blood pressure changes, diarrhoea, vaginal bleeding and headaches have been reported. Ginseng may also interact with many other medications, notably blood-thinning medications, to increase the risk of bleeding.

Clear clinical evidence for the use of ginseng as a treatment for diabetes is limited, and larger studies of better quality are required.

Yerba Maté (Ilex paraguariensis)

Obese Type 2 diabetics may be tempted to take Yerba maté to lose weight. Yerba maté is a species of holly native to subtropical South

America. Typically, the parts used are the leaf and leaf stem. Yerba maté is also known as Jesuit's tea, and is popularly drunk in Brazil, Paraguay and Argentina as a maté tea infusion, just like ordinary coffee or tea. It contains caffeine and other related substances. The usual concentration of caffeine in maté tea is 0.5–0.8%, less than in normal tea or coffee (1–2%).

Yerba maté is generally used as a stimulant to boost energy and alertness. One study[14] showed that Yerba maté could give you an earlier sense of fullness during a meal by slowing the passage of food. This could affect glucose absorption and help in weight reduction. Another study[15] showed no benefit on weight or BMI but, instead, a change in the body composition in favour of less body fat.

However, it must be noted that the caffeine in Yerba maté can contribute to insulin resistance and, thus, raise post-meal glucose level.

The caffeine in Yerba maté can also interact with many drugs, especially with excessive or prolonged intake. It can cause insomnia, restlessness, stomach upset, frequent urination and fast heart rate. Besides caffeine, Yerba maté also contains certain substances, such as tannins and N-nitroso compounds that have been linked to causing cancers. Hence, prolonged use of Yerba maté is not without risk.

Although Yerba maté's positive effect on weight and body fat composition may be compelling, there is a lack of evidence for any direct benefit on glycaemic control. This, and its potential adverse effects should make one very cautious about taking Yerba maté.

Bitter Gourd (Momordica charantia)

Bitter gourd, also known as bitter melon, balsam pear or karela, is a bitter tasting vegetable cultivated in Asia, South America and Africa.

The vegetable may contain polypeptide-P, which has similar actions to bovine insulin (insulin from cows). Other components found in bitter gourd, such as the glycoside charantin, may also lower sugar levels. Various forms have been used in diabetes, including the whole vegetable, the juice, the seeds and extracts.

It is perhaps not surprising that, amongst all botanical products that diabetics are attracted to, bitter gourd seems to command a special place. Advice on its use is usually not sought after, and if it is, most doctors do not discourage its supplementary use. The 'bitter' in its name certainly has a ring of credibility!

Although earlier clinical studies did suggest that it lowered blood sugar and enhanced the effects of conventional diabetes medications, these studies were mostly small, of short duration, non-randomised and not double-blinded[16]. A more recent, better designed study showed only 0.24% HbA1c decline with bitter gourd consumption, and even this observation was statistically weak[17].

Taking bitter gourd may cause gastrointestinal discomfort. It is also an abortifacient (substance that can induce abortion), hence it should not be used during pregnancy.

Overall, bitter gourd can be used with little risk of adverse drug effects, and may have a role in the treatment of diabetes, but the optimal amount and formulation have not been established, and more data is required.

Cinnamon Bark

Cinnamon comes from a variety of trees. Cinnamon should correctly refer to Ceylon cinnamon (*Cinnamomum verum* or C. zeylanicum), but it is found also in cassia or Chinese cinnamon (Cinnamomum aromaticum) and other species. The cinnamon commonly used as a spice may contain mixtures of extracts from these different species.

The active ingredients (e.g. polyphenolic polymer hydroxychalcone) are believed to be contained in the volatile oils from the cinnamon bark. There are some preliminary data to show that these ingredients may mimic insulin activity and improve insulin sensitivity.

Although there have been small-scale studies showing some benefit in improving blood sugar, triglyceride and cholesterol[18,19], a study in Thailand in 2006 did not show any benefits[20]. The conclusion of a recent meta-analysis[21] of five randomised controlled trials, including those cited above, was anything but positive. Diabetic people will do well *not* to replace their usual diabetes medication with cinnamon supplements. Moreover, high doses can cause contact dermatitis, oral burning sensation, stomatitis, facial flushing, vomiting and diarrhoea.

Milk Thistle (Silybum marianum)

This is a member of the aster family (which also includes daisies). There is some evidence that silymarin, the active constituent extracted from the seed, protects the liver against toxic damage, such as from alcohol.

A small 12-month study[22] in 1999 on patients with Type 2 diabetes with liver cirrhosis and on insulin showed significant improvement in glucose control when milk thistle was added, compared to insulin-only treatment. Fasting plasma glucose, HbA1c and insulin needs were lowered. More recent studies, albeit small, have also reported its efficacy in reducing blood sugar, triglyceride and cholesterol in diabetics[23,24].

Although there appears to be a role for milk thistle in poorly controlled diabetics with chronic liver disease, its routine use is still in the early stages of research. It is usually well tolerated but may cause diarrhoea, nausea, flatulence, abdominal discomfort and allergic reactions.

Fenugreek (Trigonella foenum-graecum)

This is a legume used as a spice in cooking, and is a commonly used herb in Ayurvedic and Chinese medicine. The seed powder may be mixed with food, such as *chapati*, an Indian unleavened bread.

Human clinical trials have been small and few, although published works have demonstrated that fenugreek can lower blood sugar and triglyceride, and reduce insulin resistance[25,26]. Animal studies have shown that it works by reducing carbohydrate absorption and enhancing the action of insulin.[27]

Fenugreek is generally safe when used in amounts commonly found in foods. The most common adverse side effects include diarrhoea and flatulence, abdominal pain and allergic reactions. Fenugreek may enhance the effects of anticoagulant drugs like warfarin, and blood-thinning drugs like aspirin, and thus increase the risk of bleeding. Moreover, it should not be used in pregnant women, as it may stimulate uterine contractions.

Notwithstanding the positive research data, fenugreek's role in diabetes treatment is still very preliminary.

Vanadium

This is a trace mineral which can be found in diet sources such as mushrooms, shellfish, parsley, grains, beer and wine. There is no clearly defined role for vanadium in normal body functions. Its recommended daily allowance (RDA) is not known. It is present in extremely small quantities in the blood and it cannot be measured accurately to check for deficiency. Vanadyl sulfate and sodium metavanadate are some of the common forms of vanadium used in supplements.

Vanadium is thought to mimic the actions of insulin to enhance glucose utilisation. Although more than 150 human studies on its effect on diabetes control have been published, the majority of these is small and poorly conducted[28]. Therefore, notwithstanding the handful of studies that showed positive treatment effect, vanadium cannot be currently recommended for use in diabetes. Reported adverse effects include nausea, vomiting, abdominal cramps, flatulence and diarrhoea.

Garlic (Allium sativum L.)

Garlic has been popularly used for promoting health. It has several active constituents (allicin, ajoene and allyl propyl disulfide) that are believed to have antibacterial, antioxidant, blood-thinning, sugar- and cholesterol-lowering and insulin-enhancing activities. The amount of its active constituents differs in different formulations, depending on the method of extraction. Freeze-dried garlic may contain little or no allicin.

The evidence for its health benefits is weak, at best. Two meta-analyses[29,30] showed modest effect in lowering cholesterol and preventing clotting, although a more recent study in Pakistan was more upbeat about its cholesterol-lowering benefit[31]. Another study from Russia showed that garlic tablets can lower fasting blood glucose[32]. Modest blood pressure lowering has also been shown in several studies[33].

Taking garlic supplements can cause stomach discomfort, heartburn, body odour and bad breath. Garlic, when taken with blood-thinning medications, can increase the risk of bleeding.

Garlic supplements are probably beneficial, but their blood pressure and cholesterol-lowering effects are weaker than what conventional therapies can offer. As garlic interacts with many medications, you should consult a pharmacist or doctor before taking it.

Alpha Lipoic Acid

Alpha lipoic acid (ALA) or thioctic acid is a potent antioxidant, synthesised in the liver. It is also found in foods such as liver, spinach, broccoli and potatoes. Only 30% of the amount taken from dietary or supplemental sources is absorbed. It functions as a co-factor in many enzyme complexes, and plays a part in glucose metabolism.

One of the mechanisms of diabetic complications, such as diabetic neuropathy (see Chapter 2), is tissue damage by oxygen free radicals as a result of hyperglycaemia. By being an antioxidant itself, and also by its ability to regenerate other antioxidants such as vitamin C, vitamin E and glutathione, ALA can decrease these free radicals and help thwart diabetic complications.

There have been several large clinical trials evaluating the use of ALA in diabetics. The evidence suggests that intravenous, and less so oral, ALA may relieve the pain and numbness of diabetic neuropathy[34].

ALA has good potential in the treatment of diabetic neuropathy, but more research is needed to determine the optimum dose and duration for supplementation, and whether it has any preventive potential, besides relieving symptoms. This supplement can be obtained over the counter in pharmacies. The side effects of ALA include nausea, vomiting, diarrhoea and skin rash.

EAST AND WEST

Although the use of alternative medicines and supplements occurs in all cultures and societies from time immemorial, that of traditional Eastern medicine, up to recently, had been largely empirical, and thus considered inferior and dubious.

However, many Eastern traditional medicinal and food products are being recognised as having therapeutic potential. Their full therapeutic effect awaits the outcome of their passage through the rigours of modern western scientific methods that we believe in. In this regard, Rudyard Kipling's "East is East, West is West, and never the twain shall meet" is fast becoming outdated. The best of both worlds is being harnessed for the good and enjoyment of humankind.

For now, although some of these popular alternative medicines and supplements are anecdotally efficacious in the treatment of diabetes and its complications, the approach should be one of extreme caution, as we await the results of more large, multicentre, randomised, double mask, placebo-controlled trials.

Case 31: Mr SGR – Using Diabetes Supplements

Mr SGR, a school teacher, was diagnosed with Type 2 diabetes in April 2000. His symptoms of excessive thirst and urination and a blood glucose level of 322 mg/dL (17.8 mmol/L) left no doubt about the diagnosis. He received nutritional counseling from his company dietitian while his GP treated him with metformin. Two months into the treatment he started supplementing his treatment with a tablet of 'Kordel Sugar Control' a day. As his blood sugar was subsequently in good control his GP weaned him off his metformin, as he continued with the prescribed 'diabetic diet' and the Kordel product. He soon began to experience spells of weakness, dizziness, tightness in the head and cold sweats. In one of those episodes, his blood glucose was 60 mg/dL. His symptoms would sometimes be relieved by taking sweets. When he consulted us, his HbA1c and blood glucose were normal at 5.6% and 6.1 mmol/L respectively. He was advised to stop the Kordel supplement and to continue to monitor his blood sugar before further action would be decided. Shortly after that Mr SGR went overseas for training.

Comments: It is likely that Mr SGR experienced hypoglycaemia although extreme low blood sugar was not documented. As each tablet of 'Kordel Sugar Control' contains 2 mg chromium polynicotinate (200 mcg of elemental chromium) the chromium may be the cause of the presumptive hypoglycaemia. Furthermore, it also contains 250 mg of magnesium which has been reported to have blood sugar lowering effects. While it was commendable that SGR dieted to the point of normalising his blood sugar, taking 200 mcg of chromium a day was not exactly what he needed. He did right to reveal that he was taking the supplement.

18 FREQUENTLY ASKED QUESTIONS

PART 1: ASK YOUR DIETITIAN

"We can be knowledgeable with other men's knowledge
but we cannot be wise with other men's wisdom."

—Michel de Montaigne (1533–1592)
French Renaissance thinker, writer and statesman

Q1. I don't understand why my diabetes is still not well controlled. I have switched to a vegetarian diet for the last few months.

Switching to a vegetarian diet, by itself, will not help improve your diabetic control. Controlling your diabetes includes:

- Ensuring that you have a proper understanding of your diabetes medication in relation to your diet.
- Eating the right amount and type of food at the right time.
- Having sufficient high fibre foods that can help reduce carbohydrate absorption.
- Avoiding sweet and sugary foods in your diet, unless you are experiencing hypoglycaemia.
- Exercising regularly.

Q2. Do you think I should take more vitamins, e.g. vitamin E?

If you are eating a balanced diet with sufficient fruits and vegetables in your diet, supplements are usually not necessary. However, if you are not able to eat adequate fruits and vegetables due to whatever reason, some vitamin and/or mineral supplementation may be required.

Before you do so, please check with your doctor the amount required, as taking excessive amounts, especially the fat soluble types (such as vitamin E) is not advisable.

Q3. I am taking this medicine that my friend gave me. She says the chromium in it is good for me. What do you think?

As a general rule, it is not advisable to take medication prescribed for another person, as what is good for him/her may not be suitable for you. Although chromium has been shown to reduce insulin resistance, as to whether it is good for you really depends on why you decided you need extra chromium in the first place. Do check with your doctor or pharmacist with regards to the necessity and, also, the correct amount, as too much can be harmful. The average person does not need extra chromium in his diet. If you eat a balanced diet, chances are you will not need any chromium supplement. You can get all the chromium you need from foods with a high chromium content, such as broccoli, potatoes, wholemeal muffin, grape juice, beef cubes, and orange juice.

Q4. Can I eat fruits?

Of course! Although fruits contain carbohydrates, it is good for you and necessary to provide you with vitamins, minerals and fibre. Some fruits are sweeter than others but the important thing is to have the right amount of total carbohydrate for the day. One small serving or portion of fruit (e.g. 1 slice/wedge of fruit or 1 small apple) = 10 g carbohydrate. If your dietitian has prescribed a diet of 50–60 g carbohydrate for a meal (lunch or dinner), you can always reserve 10–20 g of that allowance for fruits and make up the rest with rice, bread, potatoes or noodles. To do this, just follow the carbohydrate exchange list.

Q5. I heard that drinking red wine is good for my heart but is it suitable for diabetic patients?

The recommendations for alcohol consumption for a diabetic person is as follows:

- Abstain from drinking, where possible, especially if you do not drink in the first place. Red wine is believed to have antioxidants which protect the heart. However, you can get your antioxidants from other sources such as fruit and vegetables.
- Choose suitable alternatives such as Perrier and lime which make a nice drink without the alcohol and calories.
- If you have to, choose dry wines over sweet wines and liqueurs as the latter contain more sugar.
- For social drinking, limit yourself to one standard drink if you are a female and two standard drinks if you are a male. One standard serving means 120 ml red wine (1 wine glass). Alcohol contains sugar and provides empty calories. As such, it is not recommended if you have poor glycaemic control (e.g. blood sugar more than 10 mmol/L) and/or are overweight.
- Alcohol should be taken together with food to prevent low blood sugar.

Q6. Can I drink 'no added sugar' fruit juice?

Fruit juice contains fructose (fruit sugar). It is better to eat fresh fruits as they provide our bodies with nutrients and fibre. However, if you wish to drink fruit juice, it is recommended to drink ½ glass of unsweetened or 'no added sugar' fruit juice in place of 1 serving of fruit.

Q7. Is eating brown rice good for me?

Brown rice contains more fibre as compared to white rice, which helps to slow down blood sugar absorption. However, both brown and white rice contain the same amount of carbohydrate. Therefore, you should still control the amount of brown rice consumed.

Q8. Can I consume milk or other dairy products?

Milk and other dairy products (except cheese) contain lactose (milk sugar). Excessive intake of dairy products will affect your sugar levels. It is recommended to take about 2 servings of low-fat dairy products per day and it is preferable to select unflavoured or unsweetened varieties. You should consult your dietitian for a sample meal plan.

Q9. I love eating potatoes. As a person with diabetes, can I eat as many potatoes as I want?

The potato belongs to the starchy vegetable group (including corn, sweet potato, yam, lentils, etc.) and can affect your blood sugar levels. People with diabetes can consume potatoes in moderate amounts in place of other carbohydrate foods, such as rice, bread, noodles, etc.

Q10. Are sweeteners suitable for diabetic patients? I heard it may cause cancer.

Artificial sweeteners do not contain any sugar but some do have calories, depending on what filler has been added. (A filler is a "bulking" agent, e.g. lactose is used or added to saccharin when making artificial sweeteners.) Artificial sweeteners can be used in smaller amounts to create the same level of sweetness as sugar. The common artificial sweeteners found in the market include:

a. Those containing aspartame, commonly sold as Equal and Pal Sweet.
b. Those with sucralose, sold as Sweetico or Splenda, which has added dextrose and maltodextrin.
c. Saccharin tablets, which are not widely available. Saccharin is, however, used in many food items (e.g. preserved fruits).

The above sweeteners are regulated by the US FDA (Food and Drug Administration) and are, therefore, safe for use in moderate amounts.

Q11. I just love hawker food but now that I am a diabetic, can I eat hawker food?

Hawker food is fine as long as you know what you can eat and how much to eat. It is important that you are selective in your choice, ensuring that foods chosen are allowed in your diet and that the quantity of carbohydrate chosen is according to the prescribed amount.

Some good rules:
- Request less rice or noodles, more vegetables and less oil in the cooking. This helps to control the total amount of carbohydrate consumed for the day and also the total calories.
- Choose soup dishes instead of fried foods.
- There is no need to finish everything served if it is too much. Just eat the amount equivalent to your prescribed diet.

This way, you will not go wrong and will still get to enjoy your favourite foods, albeit occasionally!

Q12. I love to eat durians. Can I skip my meals and have durians instead?

It is definitely not a good idea, as you will not get all the nutrients your body requires from durians as compared to a balanced meal. Two seeds of durians contain about 10 g carbohydrate, the equivalent of one serving of fruit. So, if you are invited to enjoy the fruit with others, limit your intake and work out the carbohydrate portion according to your total allowance. After all, it's not worth it to over-consume and suffer the consequence of high blood sugar.

Refer also to Chapter 3, Part 2 on 'Eating Right'.

PART 2: GENERAL TOPICS

"Minds are like parachutes; they only function when they are open."

—*Sir James Dewar (1842–1923), Scottish chemist, physicist and inventor.*

FAMILY HISTORY OF DIABETES

Q1. My aunts and uncles have diabetes. I am afraid of getting diabetes too. What can I do?

Type 1 and Type 2 diabetes are, to a certain extent, hereditary but this does not mean that family members of a diabetic person will definitely get it. Of the two, Type 2 diabetes is 'more hereditary' than Type 1 diabetes. Of course, the closer you are genetically to a diabetic person, the more you are at risk.

In the case of Type 1 diabetes, the risk is relatively higher if you are a sibling of a diabetic person or if both your parents have diabetes, compared to only one parent having diabetes. Having a diabetic father puts you at a slightly higher risk than having a diabetic mother.

However, just having the diabetes genes does not automatically lead to diabetes. There is, usually, an external factor or factors that trigger it. This may be a virus infection, sedentary lifestyle or obesity.

The reality is that you cannot do anything about your genes, but you can do a lot about your lifestyle. If you are at risk because of a family history of diabetes, you should be even more careful to avoid living a sedentary lifestyle and obesity. This is particularly true of Type 2 diabetes. Furthermore, if someone in your immediate family has diabetes, you should have a screening test for diabetes once you hit 40 years old, or earlier if you have any of the other risk factors mentioned in Chapter 1.

STRESS AND DIABETES

Q2. Can stress affect my diabetes control?

Yes, in more ways than one. Many people under stress find relief from food. Your eating pattern may also become irregular, upsetting the treatment schedule. Stress hormones, such as cortisol and adrenaline from the adrenal glands, have an anti-insulin effect that raises your blood sugar.

GOING VEGETARIAN

Q3. I don't understand. I take my medicines regularly and have even switched to a vegetarian diet for the last few months. Why is my blood sugar still not controlled?

A vegetarian diet is alright but not necessarily better. Vegetable oils are generally preferred, except for coconut and palm oil, to give you a good lipid profile, but a gram of oil gives you the same calories, no matter what the source.

Where blood glucose is concerned, it is the carbohydrates that mainly affect its level, especially after a meal. Therefore, if you go vegetarian, you will still have to watch your calories and carbohydrate portions. Could it be that, as you no longer eat meat and fish, you are tucking into more carbohydrates in the form of rice, bread, potatoes and noodles? It is worth bearing in mind that carrots, although a vegetable, are also relatively high in carbohydrates.

OVERWEIGHT

Q4. Do I need to go on a special diet to reduce weight, such as the Atkins diet?

The Atkins diet is a low-carbohydrate, high-protein, high-fat diet. Fats are twice as energy dense as carbohydrates, and hence give you more calories weight for weight. One study has shown that the Atkins diet led to more weight loss compared to a conventional low calorie, high carb (carbohydrate), low-fat diet after six months, but there was no difference after a year[1]. Triglyceride level was lower and HDL-cholesterol ('good' cholesterol) was higher after the Atkins diet in this study.

Another study found that a low-carb diet also lowered the blood sugar of diabetics better than a conventional high carb, low-fat diet[2]. Yet another study showed that taking a low carb and high-fat diet raised the LDL-cholesterol ('bad' cholesterol) more[3].

Therefore, the final picture is still not very clear. The important point to remember, if you need to lose weight, is that it is all about energy balance. Aim for negative energy balance (more energy out, less energy in). And monitor your fat levels.

Q5. My doctor says that I am overweight and have pre-diabetes and he advised me to lose weight. Should I join a weight reduction programme?

If you are overweight, losing weight will, indeed, reduce your chance of developing diabetes. The most important factor is your own determination to lose weight. You can achieve this through dieting and regular exercise. Unless you already know how to achieve weight loss, it is a good idea to join a structured programme, but choose one run by sports medicine physicians, professional dietitians and exercise and fitness trainers, who will not only motivate and nudge you along but will also prescribe and supervise the appropriate diet and exercise activities that will meet your needs.

In a good centre, you can expect that your usual energy or calorie intake will be carefully calculated based on self-reporting of food intake, and a suitable diet will be recommended. Physical activities will be carefully chosen to ensure you have negative energy balance. If necessary, your resting metabolic rate can be measured to determine how much energy you expend at rest, in order to more precisely determine how many more calories you have to burn to lose weight.

FEELING HUNGRY

Q6. I have Type 2 diabetes and take glibenclamide and metformin, both twice a day. I get hungry about three hours after my breakfast and have to eat something to keep me going. My doctor says my diabetes control is not very good and I am now afraid to eat the mid-morning snack. What should I do?

Feeling hungry is not uncommon when you are on diabetes medications. It is due to the effect of the medications lowering your blood sugar. Check whether your hunger sensation is due to too much a drop in your blood sugar (i.e. hypoglycaemia). If it is, then taking a mid-morning snack is alright but discuss with your doctor whether a change of medication or dose reduction is necessary. If your hunger feeling is not associated with low blood sugar, it shows that your liver is able to break down glycogen stores to compensate for the falling blood sugar induced by the medications. You should then resist taking extra food.

Q7. I like to stay up late. Four hours after dinner I often feel hungry and I get 'gastric'. My blood sugar is not low at that time. I have no choice but to eat something. Is this alright?

The gastric pain or discomfort may be due to stomach or duodenal ulcers. If in doubt, check with your doctor or a stomach specialist. If you do not have gastro-duodenal ulcers, one way to avoid this feeling is to take more fibre with your dinner, so that the food stays in the stomach longer. Another way is to drink water to neutralise the acidic gastric juice. You do not have to resort to carbohydrate or sugar snacks, which will make your blood sugar high and undo the effects of your diabetes medicine. You can also try antacid medications to neutralise the gastric juices.

SWIMMING

Q8. I used to enjoy swimming but since starting insulin, I've been afraid to go back to the pool. What if I get a low blood glucose reaction?

Mild hypoglycaemia or low blood glucose may be a mere inconvenience, and manageable in team games, but can be dangerous when you are engaged in solitary sport activities like swimming. However, you do not have to let this stop you from swimming as long as you follow some simple safety rules:
- Do not swim if you feel unwell.
- Test your blood sugar before the swim. Proceed only when it is more than 5.5 mmol/L. Break your swim and test again if your

swimming session is long, to ensure that the blood sugar is stable. Test yet again after the swim to get an idea of its effects on your blood sugar.
- Never swim alone.
- Tell your friends or coach to get you out of the water if you behave strangely or seem to be having difficulties.
- Stop swimming immediately if you feel the first signs of a hypoglycaemia coming.
- Keep glucose tablets by the poolside for emergency treatment of hypoglycaemia.

DIABETES TABLETS

Q9. My friend told me that once I start taking anti-diabetes tablets, I will be addicted to them. I don't want to be addicted to them. What should I do?

No one, in his right mind, wants to be known as a drug addict! However, your friend's view is based on a misuse of the word 'addiction'. True drug addiction occurs when withdrawal from the drug causes psychological and physical dependence on it. Withdrawal symptoms develop if the user is deprived of the substance.

What your friend probably meant is that if you start taking diabetes tablets, you will continue to need it for the rest of your life. This is generally true. Diabetes tablets are to control your blood sugar and prevent diabetes complications. If your diabetes cannot be optimally controlled by diet and regular exercise, you will have to be treated with one or more diabetes tablets and continue on it for a long time. This is *not* addiction.

Having said that, there are patients who can reduce or go off their diabetes tablets as they take effective measures to modify their eating habits and lifestyle and lose weight (if they are overweight to start with). So, a lot also depends on your own efforts. If you want to try going off your diabetes tablets, do it gradually and only under the supervision of your doctor and with regular monitoring of your blood glucose.

Q10. Can taking diabetes medications damage my kidneys?

This is a common fear amongst many diabetic people. Diabetes medications, oral as well as insulin, are to normalise your blood glucose to prevent kidney and other complications (see Chapters 2 and 4). You probably raised this question because of a misunderstanding of what you have heard. It is when kidney failure has set in that certain diabetes medications, like metformin and glibenclamide, have to be used cautiously. Their dosage may have to be reduced or they may have to be stopped altogether. This is because the presence of kidney failure increases the risk of side effects from these medications. These medications did *not* damage your kidneys or cause kidney failure in the first place. If you have diabetes and kidney failure, the latter usually results from longstanding poor control of your diabetes and blood pressure in the first place.

Q11. I am taking oral diabetes medications. If I find that my blood glucose is high, can I take an extra dose?

It depends on many things, such as how high the blood glucose is, how you feel at that moment, what oral tablets you are taking, when was your last dose, when you are due for your next dose and meal, etc. The answer to this question has to be tailored to the individual situation. Discuss it with your diabetes care team.

INSULIN TREATMENT

Q12. I am 44 years old and overweight and have just found out that I have diabetes. My doctor has started me on insulin, and I reluctantly agreed. Is it true that if I lose weight I will not need insulin injections?

Most overweight people who have diabetes and are over 40 years old at the time of diagnosis usually have Type 2 diabetes and do not immediately need insulin. In some situations, the diabetes at the time of diagnosis may be fairly severe and requires insulin to quickly relieve symptoms and normalise the blood sugar.

You should embark on a programme of weight reduction to reduce insulin resistance. As you lose significant amounts of weight, your insulin can, usually, be gradually reduced and, eventually, stopped. So, you are right that losing weight may make it possible for your doctor to wean you off insulin. There are many factors involved in this process: how much weight you lose, how your blood sugar responds to the initial treatment and how much insulin reserve you still have from your pancreas. You would do well to get your weight to your ideal BMI and maintain it at that level. Work closely with your diabetes care team on this matter, if you want to discontinue insulin treatment, but remember that there is no guarantee that this is possible.

Q13. I am a Type 1 diabetic taking my insulin regularly, as prescribed. What should I do when I have eaten more than I should and my blood glucose is high?

First, determine what your total daily insulin dose is. Divide 1,500 by your total daily insulin dose. This will give you your insulin sensitivity index. This would then be the amount of blood glucose in *mg/dL* that will be lowered by 1 unit of insulin.

  For example:
  - Your blood glucose is 13 mmol/L and your doctor has set your ideal blood glucose at 6 mmol/L. You are therefore 7 mmol/L above the set target.
  - If your total daily insulin dose is 50 units, then your insulin index is 30 *mg/dL* (1500 ÷ 50), that is, 1 unit of insulin will lower your blood glucose by 30 *mg/dL*.
  - To convert this to mmol/L, divide by 18, hence 30 ÷ 18 = 1.6 mmol/L. To lower your blood glucose by 7 mmol/L would require about 4 additional units of insulin (7 ÷ 1.6 = 4.3).
  - Use this method only if the last insulin dose was at least four hours ago; if not, allow some time for the previous dose of insulin to work.

Q14. I am a Type 2 diabetic. If I go on insulin, do I have to take it the rest of my life?

It depends. If the need for insulin is because all else have failed, then your diabetes has progressed to such a state that you will have to take insulin for the rest of your life. There are, however, some situations when your insulin dose can be reduced or stopped or when you need it only for a short term:

Firstly, if, despite the best efforts, including insulin treatment, kidney failure has developed, insulin dosage can sometimes be reduced or even stopped. This is actually not a desirable situation, because it means that your kidney failure is fairly advanced. Stopping insulin in this situation is possible only when your pancreas is still making some insulin. Now, besides the liver, the kidneys also participate in the breakdown of insulin. If the kidneys are not functioning well, they break down less insulin. Therefore, ironically, you may now have 'enough' of your own insulin and do not need insulin injections.

Secondly, if you have Type 2 diabetes and have been put on insulin because of an episode of diabetic ketoacidosis or hyperosmolar hyperglycaemia syndrome, insulin may be stopped when this acute complication has resolved, but do not do so without first consulting your doctor.

Thirdly, if you are obese, and have started taking insulin because your diabetes is severe and you have lots of symptoms, as you lose weight through dieting and exercise, you may be able to go off insulin and just take diabetes tablets (see Question 12 above).

Fourthly, insulin is very often used in Type 2 diabetics to tighten their sugar control in preparation for major surgery. In this situation, you can go off insulin when you have recovered from the surgery.

Fifthly, insulin is necessary on a short-term basis during an acute stress event such as a heart attack, infection or injury.

Lastly, insulin may be necessary during pregnancy but not necessary after the birth of the child, if control is good without it (see Chapter 12).

Q15. I have been taking insulin for so long. Will there be any problem?

Your intended meaning is whether there are any long-term side effects to taking insulin. The main purpose of using insulin is to lower the blood glucose. Indeed, you can get an 'over effect' if the dose is too much for your needs, causing hypoglycaemia or low blood glucose. This can happen if you reduce your food intake, miss a meal or increase your physical activity. It can also happen if you develop kidney failure.

Another side effect of insulin is weight gain. If you have Type 1 diabetes and have lost weight as a result of it, gaining weight is what you need. If you have Type 2 diabetes and are already overweight, but need insulin because oral tablets are no longer working, then the weight gain may not be so welcome. However, the benefits of having normal glucose levels outweigh the disadvantage of weight gain. To minimise the weight gain, work harder on your diet and exercise so that the insulin dose can be kept to the minimum.

Insulin repeatedly injected into a small area of your body can cause fat accumulation (insulin lipohypertrophy) and hardening of that area. Insulin injected into such a lipohypertrophied area is absorbed erratically and might cause difficulty in control. Hence, always change the spot at which you give the injection.

Q16. Is it dangerous to inject air bubbles that may be trapped in the syringe after drawing out the insulin?

Tiny air bubbles, even when introduced into a vein, are quickly dispersed and are unlikely to do any harm. On the other hand, very large amounts of air injected into the bloodstream could be dangerous. However, these amounts are far larger than what could be trapped in the insulin syringe. The main reason for getting rid of air bubbles in your syringe before injection is that air bubbles take up space and you may end up injecting less insulin than you should.

Q17. What should I do if I suddenly realise that I have missed my insulin injection?

Occasionally, you may forget to give yourself insulin or, even worse, forget whether you have already taken the insulin. When this happens, you should check your blood sugar to help you decide what you should do next. If your blood glucose is high (more than 10 mmol/L), it is likely you have forgotten to give your injection and should inject your insulin immediately. If your blood sugar is normal or low (5 mmol/L or less), you have probably taken your insulin and could have forgotten that you have done so. It is best to check your blood glucose again before your next meal. If the level is high, inject an extra dose of short-acting insulin.

SELF BLOOD GLUCOSE MONITORING

Q18. How often do I have to check my blood sugar?

There is no hard and fast rule. It depends on the individual situation. A pregnant woman should check seven times a day, three to four days a week, and the majority do so without complaining. On the other hand, the stable Type 2 diabetic, on single pill therapy and living a fairly uniform daily routine, may only need to do a test once a week, just to be sure that everything is alright. Your doctor or diabetes nurse clinician will advise you on this. See also Chapter 5.

Bear in mind that checking your blood sugar at home, at work and even when travelling is the only way you can understand how meals, activities and medications affect your blood glucose levels. The more you test, the more you understand these complex interactions. Moreover, test at different times of the day and do not restrict testing to just a fasting pre-breakfast test, so that you get an overall and more complete idea of your blood sugar during the day. It is like when you want to appreciate a big painting, you don't just focus on one corner of the painting!

HIGH BLOOD GLUCOSE (HYPERGLYCAEMIA)

Q19. I am a Type 2 diabetic who, unfortunately, requires insulin. I am taking Insulatard before breakfast and before dinner, in addition to gliclazide and metformin twice a day. My doctor said I am doing okay, as my HbA1c is 7.2% and fasting blood sugar is 5–6 mmol/L. However, I notice that, without fail, two hours after my breakfast, my blood sugar is always higher than 10 mmol/L and will only come down much later, although I don't think my breakfast is too heavy. How can I get a lower blood sugar two hours after my breakfast?

You brought up an interesting observation. Yes, there is general agreement amongst diabetes specialists, that, besides the HbA1c and the fasting blood glucose, the after-meal blood glucose should, ideally, be as normal as possible (6–8 mmol/L) to prevent damage to blood vessels.

What you are experiencing is probably because both your insulin (Insulatard®) and gliclazide have not started to work to the maximum two hours after your breakfast. One way to improve the situation is to replace your gliclazide with an alternative that works faster, such as replaglinide or nateglinide. This has to be taken 5–10 minutes before your breakfast, as it starts to act within that time. Its action peaks 1–2 hours after you take it. However, its action lasts only 4–5 hours and, therefore, you will have to take it three times a day before each meal, unlike gliclazide, which acts slower but lasts longer and can be taken twice a day. Your question illustrates that the treatment of diabetes has to be individualised.

Q20. This morning, my fasting blood glucose at home was 7 (mmol/L). Why is it 8.2 here at the hospital? I haven't eaten anything yet.

Assuming you have done the test correctly and your glucometer is in good working condition, one reason could be that the effect of the previous day's or night's oral medications and/or insulin are wearing off with time. Another reason could be that your glucose meter may not be the same type as your doctor's or the hospital's. Or it could be the way the blood glucose is measured in the hospital. In many hospital laboratories, blood glucose is measured as *plasma* glucose, which is 10–15% higher than *whole blood* glucose (finger-prick meter-based tests measure whole blood glucose). Furthermore, many hormones in our body have a diurnal variation, meaning that their levels are not the same from midnight to dawn compared to later in the day. Cortisol, a stress hormone produced by the adrenal glands, in particular, gradually rises as the morning progresses. This hormone counters the action of insulin, and hence your blood glucose may be higher at the clinic two hours after your test at home.

Q21. Why is my fasting blood glucose higher than my bedtime blood glucose? I was sleeping the whole night and did not wake up in the middle of the night to eat anything.

Our body needs to have glucose all the time, even when we seem to be doing nothing but sleeping. During the night, although no food is eaten after dinner, the liver ensures that there is enough sugar in our blood to keep us alive. It makes glucose (a process called gluconeogenesis) and releases it into the bloodstream.

When your blood sugar in the morning is higher than when you went to sleep, there could be a number of reasons. When you have diabetes, gluconeogenesis continues uninhibited, because of either the lack of insulin, or insulin resistance, or both. Therefore, the situation that you encounter calls for an adjustment of your treatment. This may require an increase in the dose of your oral medications or, in particular, the evening dose of insulin (if you are on it).

LOW BLOOD GLUCOSE (HYPOGLYCAEMIA)

Q22. I have been a Type 1 diabetic for 36 years on twice daily intermediate- and regular short-acting insulin. My HbA1c is 6.9% but I think I am getting 'hypo' in the middle of the night, as I sometimes sweat profusely. My blood sugar must be quite low as I do not get 'hypo' symptoms until my blood glucose is less than 3.2 (mmol/L). What should I do?

Nocturnal 'hypo' occurs for a number of reasons, such as too much pre-dinner intermediate-acting insulin, too little carbohydrates for dinner or excessive exercise during the day. If you are not already overweight, taking a bedtime snack would usually solve the problem, especially if you have had a lot of physical activity during the day. Or you could reduce the pre-dinner intermediate insulin.

Discuss this with your diabetes care team. Sometimes, injecting the intermediate-acting insulin at bedtime, instead of before dinner; or changing to a peakless long-acting insulin (such as insulin glargine or insulin detemir) at bedtime, in place of the pre-dinner intermediate-acting insulin, might help.

Not being able to get warning symptoms of a 'hypo' is common in longstanding diabetes and it can be dangerous. This is called 'hypo unawareness'. One solution that your doctor might try is to reduce your insulin dose to allow your blood glucose to rise a little; you will soon find that symptoms of 'hypo' will be experienced at a higher blood glucose level (say, 4 mmol/L) to warn you to take a snack before it gets worse.

WHEN HAVING A FLU

Q23. I recently had a flu and was given various medicines, including cough medicine and antibiotics. My blood sugar was higher than usual during that period, till I recovered from the illness. I did not take my diabetes medicine regularly then, as I was taking so many other medicines. The cough syrup was very sweet. What should I do the next time I have the same illness?

Common flu medicine can be taken with oral diabetes medicine and insulin. It is very unlikely that the high blood sugar level was due to the cough medicine, since a dose of cough syrup contains only 5 g of sugar. It is more likely that the illness itself raised your blood sugar level because of the stress hormones released in response to the illness. (If you are concerned the next time you have a flu, request sugar-free cough syrup.) When you have a flu or any acute illness, you should continue to take your usual diabetes medications and check your blood glucose more frequently. Not taking your usual diabetes medicine can be dangerous. (See Case 19, Chapter 7.) You usually need to step up the dose of diabetes medicine unless your diabetes has been in superb control and you are not eating much at all. Even then, do not guess your blood sugar level, but instead check it more frequently and check your urine for the presence of ketones if the blood glucose is above 15 mmol/L. If the urine tests positive for ketones, call or see your doctor as soon as possible before you develop diabetic ketoacidosis (See Chapter 2).

RETINOPATHY

Q24. My eye doctor advised me to have laser treatment for my diabetic retinopathy. I am afraid of laser therapy. My friend, who is also a diabetic, had laser therapy and his eyesight became worse. What should I do?

Your friend may have had worse retinopathy to start with, or may have started laser treatment too late to benefit much from it. Laser therapy is safe and effective. It destroys the damaged areas in your retina and reduces the risk of sudden bleeding in the retina. It is painless, although some patients report a mild, temporary discomfort. Laser therapy may sometimes not improve the condition, but it will stabilise and slow down the worsening of vision. Therefore, although there may be some discomfort after the laser treatment or even a slight deterioration of your vision, you are less likely to suffer a major catastrophe.

TRAVEL

Q25. Is it safe for someone with diabetes to take travel sickness tablets?

Travel sickness tablets should not upset diabetes control. However, they may make you sleepy, so be careful if you are driving. This sleepiness may be confused with hypoglycaemia. On the other hand, vomiting from motion sickness can destabilise your diabetes control; therefore it is advisable to take travel sickness tablets to prevent motion sickness if you are prone to it.

Q26. I am going on an overseas holiday for just one week. Can I take tablets instead of my usual insulin?

No, never ever think of it! If you need insulin in the first place, it is not advisable to replace your insulin with oral medications, even for a few days. Blood glucose can rise very quickly and spoil your holiday. Many instances of diabetic ketoacidosis and hyperosmolar hyperglycaemia syndrome (see Chapter 2) are due to skipping insulin. In fact, you should ensure that you have enough insulin when abroad, and carry your insulin in your hand luggage, so that, should you lose your checked-in luggage, you will not be stranded without insulin.

HORMONE REPLACEMENT THERAPY

Q27. I would like to know if hormone replacement therapy for menopause is suitable for people with diabetes.

Hormone replacement therapy (HRT) is given to menopausal women who are experiencing unpleasant symptoms like hot flushes. In the past, it was considered safe as long as you do not have pre-existing heart disease, stroke, high blood pressure, thrombosis, liver disease or gallstones, but, in recent years, it has been found that HRT with pills containing both oestrogen and progesterone could increase the risk of heart disease and breast cancer. The pros and cons of HRT have to be weighed carefully. Your doctor is the best person to decide if you need hormone replacement therapy. HRT may affect diabetes control. If you are on HRT and have diabetes, monitor your blood sugar more frequently during the first three months after starting on HRT.

19 THE FUTURE

"The future belongs to those who see possibilities
before they become obvious."

—*John Sculley (1939–)*
American businessman, former president of PepsiCo and CEO of Apple Computer.

YOUR FOREMOST QUESTION

The foremost and final question in your mind must be: "When will a cure for diabetes come?" Indeed, where is diabetes heading? What does the future hold for the patient? When can he or she not have to take diabetes tablets, insulin injections and prick fingers to test blood sugar?

Seeing the Future through the Past

Since the discovery of animal source insulin in 1921 and the advent of longer-acting insulins and oral diabetes medicines in the 1950s, there has been a relentless search for better medicine and diagnostic and therapeutic tools, and the ultimate—a cure. Hence, the portable glucose meter was developed in the late 1970s, HbA1c test and human insulin appeared in the 1980s, and insulin analogues in the 1990s. The battle is slowly being won, to make living with diabetes more bearable.

Blood Glucose Monitoring Aids[1]

An intense race is on to make non-invasive or minimally invasive instruments for blood glucose tests that do not require blood-letting or finger-pricking. Some of the technology used includes the use of infra-red, ultrasound and electromagnetic sensing. Only a handful have met the stringent rules of regulatory bodies and some, having been approved, have subsequently been removed from the market. Here are two that have made it:

The Lasette Laser Lancing Device (Cell Robotics) is a device that draws a drop of blood using laser (instead of the usual lancet), making a small hole, almost painlessly, in the skin of your fingertip. It has been approved by the US FDA. Its drawback is that it is much bigger than the average lancet-dependent finger-pricking device and it comes with a hefty price tag.

GlucoWatch Biographer (Cygnus Inc, USA) has also received approval from the US FDA. This device is worn like a wristwatch. Using a small current, fluid from under the skin is extracted for glucose measurement. It can show up to three glucose readings an hour for 12 hours, giving you the blood glucose trend for detecting and evaluating episodes of high or low blood glucose. However, the results from this 'watch' have to be confirmed by blood-based conventional glucose meters before you take corrective action.

FOUR NEW DIRECTIONS IN DIABETES DRUG DEVELOPMENT

The selection of the following four new directions for comment is *absolutely arbitrary*. There is no rationale to choose them over countless other paths, except to reiterate and illustrate the innovativeness of scientists in their quest for better and complementary drugs. They are just a small sampling from a vast research field that boggles the minds of even the well-read.

As mentioned in Chapter 1, one of the hormones that play an important role in keeping our blood sugar stable is glucagon. Glucagon has actions that are generally opposite to those of insulin. Researchers are working on chemical agents that oppose the actions of glucagon. These glucagon antagonists[2] reduce glucose production by the liver during the fasting state and store up the glucose as glycogen instead, thereby lowering blood sugar.

Others are looking at the complex biochemical steps in the beta cells by which glucose is processed, leading to the synthesis and secretion of insulin, and the way glucose is converted into storage glycogen in the liver. One of the key enzymes involved in these processes is glucokinase. Conceivably, if we can enhance the action of this enzyme, we can increase insulin production and store up more glucose as glycogen. Indeed, animal studies on glucokinase *activators*[2] have shown promising results in increasing insulin levels, converting more glucose into glycogen and, ultimately, lowering blood sugar. Studies on glucokinase activators have moved into early clinical phases.

In diabetes, as mentioned in Chapter 1, when the blood glucose is high, glucose passes through the filtering apparatus of the kidneys to be excreted in the urine. There is a transporter system in the kidneys that will reabsorb some of this filtered glucose. Scientists are studying a novel group of drugs that inhibit this transporter system so that more glucose is passed out in the urine. Preliminary clinical trials have, indeed, shown that these drugs reduce blood glucose and promote weight loss as more glucose is excreted.[3] Although they do not target the basic defects in diabetes, they are potentially useful add-on drugs to current medications.

To round up, it has been observed that caloric restriction reduces diseases of aging, including Type 2 diabetes, cataracts, cancers and atherosclerosis. Enzymes called sirtuins, widely distributed in the body, are believed to mediate the effects of caloric restriction. A group of compounds, called sirtuin-activating compounds (SRACs)[2], turn on these sirtuins. They are currently being tested to verify their role in lowering blood glucose and other health benefits.

The future will definitely throw up more candidate diabetes drugs. Many will fall by the wayside while others will survive for a while. A few will be real breakthroughs. Look out for news and views, but beware of media hypes and always read them in context.

IS A CURE IN SIGHT?

The crystal ball is not entirely clear. Work on a cure is focused on five major areas.

The Artificial Pancreas

We have mentioned two relatively recent innovations: the insulin pump in Chapter 3 Part 5 and the continuous glucose monitoring system or CGMS in Chapter 5.

The functions of insulin pumps are ever expanding. Some new models can be programmed to calculate how much insulin you need for a given meal and the prevailing blood glucose. However, you still need to prick your finger for the blood glucose reading and activate the insulin pump to deliver the insulin. More advanced models incorporate the CGMS. The latter shows you real-time blood glucose as well as its trend in the preceding 24 hours in the form of a graph, to help you decide on the dose of insulin you need. You do not have to prick your finger to obtain your blood glucose level, but you still have to manually activate the pump to deliver the requisite insulin.

At Cambridge University, 'finishing touches' are being done to refine a computerised algorithm to 'close the loop' between the insulin pump and the CGMS. The algorithm will enable the pump to use the glucose sent in by the CGMS to deliver the appropriate dose of insulin without conscious effort from you, thus creating the artificial pancreas.

Another version of the artificial pancreas is being developed, notably in France. This experimental device uses a blood glucose sensor placed in the jugular vein, a blood vessel in the neck that leads to the heart. The sensor is connected by a transmitter line placed under the skin to an implanted insulin pump. The glucose sensor instructs the pump, via a computerised algorithm, to deliver the appropriate dose of insulin to keep the blood sugar normal.

Pancreas Transplant

Although transplantation of pancreas using cadaveric donors has been around since the 1960s, it is still considered experimental. Nonetheless, it is becoming more accepted and offered as a viable option as results are improving with better surgical techniques, more effective immunosuppressive anti-rejection drugs and better post-surgical care. Patient survival of more than 95%, graft survival of more than 80%, and an improved quality of life can be expected.[4]

Pancreas transplant can be done for Type 1 diabetics or Type 2 diabetics who require insulin shortly after diagnosis and whose risk of diabetic complications outweighs the risk of transplant and anti-rejection therapy.

The majority of pancreas transplants are simultaneous pancreas and kidney transplant (SPK) as opposed to pancreas transplant alone (PTA) and pancreas after kidney transplant (PAK), although the latter two are becoming more popular.

Patients have to be carefully selected and thoroughly evaluated to give them the best possible outcome. This form of therapy is restricted by the availability of expertise and the lack of donors.

Islet Cell Transplant

The islet cells of the pancreas, you will remember, are the source of insulin. Islet cell transplant is being done in several renowned diabetes centres, but the technique and protocol used in the University of Alberta, Edmonton, Canada since 2001 is, by far, the most often cited for the long-term viability of this approach.

Islet cells from cadaveric donors are processed, purified and injected into the livers of carefully selected Type 1 diabetics, who are then treated with non-steroid anti-rejection drugs. The actual injection administration of the islets can be done on an outpatient basis.

Although about 60% of patients thus treated could go off insulin at one point after the treatment, three quarters of these patients needed insulin again within two years. The good news is that those who still needed insulin after the transplant needed a smaller dose than before the transplant and had fewer fluctuations in blood sugar levels

Hence, islet cell transplant is only partially successful. The future lies in the development of more effective anti-rejection drugs with fewer toxic effects and in overcoming the shortage of donor islet cells.

Stem Cell Therapy

In theory, stem cells (which are early cells that have not yet differentiated into any specific tissue or organ) can be made to develop into islet cells that can make insulin. In current research, either adult or embryonic stem cells are 'coaxed' towards this end.

Adult stem cells are relatively more differentiated and, theoretically, easier to develop along the desired cell line, but they cannot reproduce as easily. On the other hand, embryo stem cells can reproduce faster but, being developmentally much earlier cells that have the potential to develop into more organs, it is harder to make them develop specifically into insulin producing cells.

To date, fully functional islets have not yet been derived from stem cells. Hope was raised in 2007 when stem cell therapy in a small group of newly diagnosed Type 1 diabetics in the USA and Brazil led to varying periods of freedom from insulin. Experts, however, were quick to caution that it was too early to celebrate.

Gene Therapy

Scientists are researching the use of genes to prevent and treat various diseases, including diabetes. The principle of gene therapy is based on the insertion of genes to replace, alter or supplement missing or defective genes associated with the disease.

Diabetes with single-gene defects, such as the rare form called Maturity Onset Diabetes of the Young (MODY) (see Chapter 1), are more amenable to such treatment. However, the majority of diabetics have either Type 1 or Type 2 diabetes, in which many genes and environmental factors are involved. They are, therefore, less amenable to gene replacement, but that is not stopping the adventurous from going all out to identify these culprit genes and find ways to fix them.

Gene therapy research is also focusing heavily on stimulating insulin and insulin-producing beta cells and disabling the immune system that destroys beta cells in Type 1 diabetes. Other work focuses on treating diabetic complications, such as diabetic neuropathy, diabetic foot ulcers and even erectile dysfunction. Yet others are exploring ways to use genes to get non-beta cells to produce insulin, thus outsmarting the runaway immune system that destroys beta cells in Type 1 diabetes.

In gene therapy, a carrier, or vector, is used to deliver genes into a tissue or organ. The vector is either a virus that has been rendered harmless, or a non-viral material, such as a protein, a synthetic lipid shell or plasmids (DNA molecules from bacteria).

In in-vivo gene therapy, the healthy or modified gene is introduced directly into the body. In contrast, ex-vivo (or in-vitro) gene therapy involves taking out the subject's gene, modifying it outside the body and placing it back into the patient.

Gene therapy in diabetes is still experimental. Most of the current research is conducted on animals with few human clinical trials. Problems that have not been solved include infection from the viral vector, immune reaction to the viral vector, and inadvertent over-production of insulin by non-beta cells that have been transfected with insulin-making genes.

Although it is still early days, the potential of a cure of diabetes by gene therapy cannot be dismissed.

Of the five areas, the artificial pancreas holds the most promise, as it is likely to be the most widely available in the foreseeable future. Pancreas and islet cell transplants have been generally successful but are limited by shortage of expertise and donor pancreases and islet cells.

THE BIG PICTURE

It is obvious that, in discussing research and the future, we have not touched on the 'softer' issues of diabetes care. Much is continually being studied and learnt about issues such as who are more prone to get diabetes, who are more prone to or protected from diabetic complications, the psychosocial implications of diabetes, the pedagogy or science of diabetes education, etc., just to sample a tiny drop from a vast ocean. Such studies may not directly lead to a cure, but are important in enhancing our understanding of diabetes and teaching us how to manage it now and in the future.

THE FUTURE IS EVERYBODY'S BUSINESS

Although we have been discussing topics that are the domain of those who have a special or specific calling, the future of diabetes care should be everybody's concern.

Greater awareness of the risk factors of the disease should make us all lead a healthier lifestyle. At the state and community level, there should not be any let up in promoting disease awareness, implementing preventive measures and providing comprehensive primary, secondary and tertiary care. There should be societal and administrative resolve and resources to minimise exposing the population to unhealthy food and to provide facilities to encourage regular exercise. Diabetes drugs and management tools should be made more affordable to all diabetic people and be affordably covered by insurance. The results of diabetes research should be harnessed judiciously for the benefit of the patients.

Not putting in enough effort would result in heavy human attrition and a drain on different economies as populations age and more succumb to diabetes around the world.

20 CONCLUSION

Although we have good reasons to look to the future with optimism and hope, it behoves us to come full circle and constantly remind ourselves that patient education in diabetes self-care is integral to good diabetes management.

At the end of this short walk with our *Diabetes Companion*, there are choices to make. Increasingly, you, who have diabetes, are being empowered to take charge. There are many ways you can equip yourself with the knowledge and skills to help you in the journey ahead. In this regard, there is no shortage of educational material and resources, of which this humble book is but one.

Together with your diabetes care team, you are in life's constant drama, where you are the lead actor or actress and the rest of us are, at best, directors, supporting players, musicians, orchestra conductors, script writers, stage crew, costume designers, etc. The audience is waiting to applaud you. The show must go on till the final curtain comes down on an enigmatic play that you did not choose to be a part of, but, nevertheless, has become a part of you.

The end is not yet in sight, but, with the rapid advances in diabetes research, and with people around you cheering you on, it is vital that you keep yourself as healthy as possible as you wait patiently for a cure, so that you can seize the moment when it comes.

"I never see what has been done,
I only see what remains to be done."

—*Marie Curie (1867–1934), French-Polish physicist*
twice-honoured Nobel Laureate

LIST OF CASES

GLOSSARY OF MEDICAL JARGON

A1c	Short for HbA1c (see HbA1c).
ACE-inhibitors	Angiotensin converting enzyme inhibitors, a class of drugs for treating high blood pressure.
Adipose tissues	Fat or fatty tissues.
Aerobic exercise	Exercise, using large muscles, that requires and increases oxygen consumption for sustained periods.
Amino acids	The component units of protein.
Anaerobic exercise	Also called resistance exercise. It uses large muscles which do not require oxygen for short periods of exercise.
Analogue	A chemical similar in structure to another but differing from it in some components to either enhance its action or produce an opposite effect.
Antioxidant	Substances, natural or synthetic, used to prevent oxidation of another substance, and thereby prevent damage produced by free radicals, which are products of oxidation. See Free Radicals.
ARBs	Angiotensin receptor blockers; a class of drugs used to treat hypertension.
Aromatherapy	A form of alternative medicine that uses volatile liquid plant materials, known as essential oils, and other aromatic compounds from plants for the purpose of affecting a person's mood or health.
Atherosclerosis	Hardening and thickening of arteries due to deposition of plaques containing cholesterol, among other substances. It is the commonest underlying cause of cardiovascular disease (see definition in this Glossary).
Autonomic neuropathy	Disease of the autonomic nerves.
Ayurvedic medicine	A form of Indian or Hindu medicine.
Bariatric surgery	Surgery for the treatment of overweight. (Bariatry is the study of overweight: its causes, prevention and treatment.)

Bile	An alkaline golden brown to greenish fluid secreted by the liver into the small intestines.
BMI	Body mass index, a measure of degree of obesity.
Calorie	Unit of heat energy. A calorie or cal. is the amount of heat energy needed to raise 1 kilogram of water by 1 degree Celcius at a specified temperature. In nutrition, 1 kilocalorie (formerly written as Calorie, that is with a big "C") is now simply written as 1 calorie (that is, with a small "c").
Carbohydrate	Compounds consisting of carbon, hydrogen and oxygen that function as sources of energy. They include sugar (simple carbohydrates) and starches (complex carbohydrates).
Cardiovascular disease (CVD)	Disease of the arteries characterised by diminished blood flow leading to coronary artery disease, cerebral thrombosis/thrombotic stroke and peripheral arterial disease (see respective definitions in this glossary).
Cardiac neuropathy	Dysfunction of the heart due to neuropathy (see Neuropathy).
Cataract	Opacity of the eye lens causing blurring of vision.
Cerebral thrombosis	Clot formation in the cerebral arteries leading to reduced blood flow and thrombotic stroke.
Cholesterol	Chemically a wax-like substance that is found in food and also produced in the liver. It is a key constituent of cell membranes and can accumulate or deposit in gallstones and the inner lining of arteries causing blockage and reducing blood flow.
Cochrane database	A source of high quality data from the Cochrane Library on medical research and reviews. It is recognised as the gold standard in evidence-based health care.
Co-factor	A substance with which another must unite in order to function.
Coronary artery disease (CAD)	Refers to blockage of the coronary arteries which supply blood to the the heart muscles.
Coronary heart disease	Heart disease due to CAD (see definition in this Glossary).
Dermatitis	Inflammation of the skin.
Diabetes Insipidus	A disease due to insufficient production of a hormone called vasopressin. It is unrelated to diabetes mellitus.
Diabetic Ketoacidosis (DKA)	An acute complication of diabetes due to severe insulin lack and characterised by high blood glucose and ketones, dehydration and breathlessness.

Diabetic nephropathy	Kidney disease due to diabetes.
Diabetic neuropathy	Nerve disease or damage due to diabetes.
Diabetic retinopathy	Diseases of the retina due to diabetes.
Dialysis (renal)	The process by which macromolecules (waste materials) are removed from the blood through a semi-permeable membrane.
Double mask	Pertaining to clinical trials and other experiments in which both the subject and the person conducting the experiment do not know which drug treatment the subject is receiving. Also known as double blind.
Erectile Dysfunction	Impairment of erection of the penis.
Essential amino acids	Amino acids required for protein synthesis that are not produced by the human and, therefore, have to be obtained from food sources. There are nine such amino acids.
Exudates (retinal)	Material such as fluid, cells, cell debris, which have passed from blood vessel on to tissues or to their surfaces.
Free radicals	Radicals (groups of atoms that participate in chemical reactions without change) that carry unpaired electrons and which are injurious to cells.
Gangrene	Death of viable tissue due to lack of blood supply.
Gestational diabetes mellitus (GDM)	Diabetes occurring or diagnosed during pregnancy.
Glaucoma	A group of eye diseases characterised by increased pressure in the eyeball, potentially causing blurring of vision.
Glucagon	A hormone secreted by the islets of Langerhans in the pancreas in close proximity to insulin-producing cells. It has effects on blood glucose and metabolism opposite to those of insulin.
Gluconeogenesis	The formation of glucose from substances that are not themselves carbohydrates, such as amino acids.
Glucose	A simple carbohydrate present in fruits and plants and in the blood of all animals. It is the primary source of energy in animals. See also 'Sugar' and 'Carbohydrates' in this Glossary.
Glycated haemoglobin	Haemoglobin (the red pigments in the red blood cells that carry oxygen) that are tagged with simple sugars, such as glucose.
Glycogen	The storage form of excess glucose found primarily in the liver and muscles.

Glycosuria	The presence of glucose in the urine.
HbA1c	Stands for haemoglobin A1c, the major form of glycated haemoglobin (refer to this word in this Glossary).
HDL-cholesterol	High-density-lipoprotein cholesterol or the so-called 'good cholesterol' because it reflects the cholesterol taken up from the peripheral tissues, such as the walls of blood vessels, and transported to the liver for excretion in the bile.
Homeopathic	Pertaining to a system of therapeutics in alternative medicine that uses small amounts of drugs that normally produce, in healthy people, the very symptoms of the disease it seeks to cure.
Hormones	Chemical substances produced by organs (especially the glands), e.g. the pancreas, having specific regulatory effects on the activity of an organ or organs, e.g. the liver and the muscles.
Hyperglycaemia	High blood glucose.
Hyperosmolar Hyperglycaemic Syndrome (HHS)	An acute complication of diabetes due to severe insulin lack, characterised by high blood glucose and severe dehydration.
Hypertension	High blood pressure.
Hypoglycaemia	Low blood glucose.
Hypoglycaemia unawareness	Unawareness of the presence of hypoglycaemia because of the absence of the typical symptoms.
Immunosuppressive	That which suppresses the immune system.
Incretins	Hormones produced by specific cells in the small intestines, having multiple actions, predominantly the secretion of insulin and suppression of glucagon in the presence of high blood glucose.
Insulin	A hormone produced by the beta-cells of the islets of Langerhans of the pancreas, with predominant actions on the metabolism of carbohydrate, protein and fats.
Insulin analogues	Insulin molecules that have been modified to alter their chemical and physical properties for use in the treatment of diabetes.
Insulin lipohypertrophy	Localised hypertrophy (increase in size) of the site of insulin injection due to accumulation of fat.
Insulin receptors	Molecules on the surface membranes of cells that react with insulin to allow glucose to enter the cells.
Insulin secretagogues	A drug that stimulate the beta-cells in the islets of Langerhans to produce and release insulin.

Insulin sensitivity index	The approximate amount of blood glucose (in terms of concentration) that can be reduced by 1 unit of insulin based on a formula of calculation.
Interstitial fluid	The fluid in the space between cells and outside of the blood vessels.
Ischaemia or ischaemic	Ischaemia is deprivation or deficiency of blood supply, and 'ischaemic' is the adjective derived thereof.
Islets of Langerhans	Clusters of cells in the pancreas in which specialised alpha-cells produce the hormone glucagon, beta-cells produce insulin and delta-cells produce somatostatin.
Ketones	Incomplete breakdown products of fats.
Ketosis	Abnormally high levels of ketones in body fluid, such as blood.
Lactose	A simple carbohydrate which is the major constituent of mammalian milk.
LADA	Latent Autoimmune Diabetes of Adults.
Laser surgery or photocoagulation	The use of laser to burn and eradicate parts of the retina that are deprived of blood supply, and thus prevent formation of fragile new vessels that bleed easily.
Lipids	A group of substances that include fat and fat-like substances, such as neutral fats (triglyceride), fatty acids and cholesterol.
Lipid profile	The concentration of lipids in the blood. It typically includes the total cholesterol, HDL-cholesterol, LDL-cholesterol, triglyceride and the total cholesterol to HDL-cholesterol ratio.
Lipoproteins	Organic complexes in which lipids (cholesterol and triglyceride) are transported in the bloodstream.
Low-density lipoprotein cholesterol	It is the so-called 'bad cholesterol', as it represents the cholesterol transported to the peripheral tissues, including the walls of blood vessels where it forms deposits and plaques.
Macroalbuminuria	The presence of albumin, a protein, in the urine with a concentration high enough to be measured by conventional means, often due to diabetes.
Macrosomia	Abnormally large size.
Macula retinae	A small area on the retina that absorbs short wavelengths of light.
Macular oedema	Swelling of the macula retinae of the retina, causing blurring of vision.
Maculopathy	Disease of the macula retinae.

Meta-analysis	Systematic method that uses statistical analysis to integrate the data from a number of independent studies.
Metabolism	The sum of all the physical and chemical processes that produce and maintain the living organism (anabolism) and also the breakdown of substances to produce energy (catabolism) for use by the organism.
mg/dL	Milligram per deciliter, a non-metric unit of measurement of the concentration of a substance in fluid, such as blood.
Microalbuminuria	The presence of albumin, a protein, in the urine with concentration higher than normal but too subtle to be measured by conventional means, often due to diabetes. See Macroalbuminuria.
Microaneurysm	Small sac formed by expansion of a small blood vessel.
Micronutrients	Essential dietary substances required only in trace amounts. Examples: vitamins and minerals (phosphorus, iodine, magnesium, etc).
mmol/L	Millimole per litre, a metric unit of measurement of the concentration of a substance in the fluid, such as blood.
Monounsaturated fats (fatty acids)	Fats in which the fatty acids have only one double bond (between carbon units). They occur predominantly in certain vegetable and seed oils.
Neovascularisation (retinal)	Formation of new blood vessels on the retina in response to deprivation of normal blood supply.
Nephropathy	Disease of the kidneys.
Neuropathy	Disease of the nerves.
Neutral fat	A compound of glycerol and fatty acids. Also referred to as triglyceride.
Non-aerobic exercise	Exercise that does not increase oxygen consumption.
Omega-3 and omega-6 fatty acids	Certain types of unsaturated fats found predominantly in certain fish, vegetables and seeds, with the effect of lowering triglyceride and increasing levels of HDL-cholesterol.
Pancreas	An elongated organ that produces digestive enzymes as well hormones, such as insulin and glucagon, situated in the abdomen just below and behind the stomach.
Peripheral neuropathy	Damage of the peripheral nerves, i.e. nerves that supply organs and structure near the surface of the body, such as muscles, skin and sweat glands.
Peripheral vascular disease	Diseases of the arteries that decrease the supply of blood to superficial structures, such as skin and muscles.

Phospolipids	Any lipid that contains phosphorus. Phospholipids are the major form of lipids in all cell membranes.
Placenta	A foeto-maternal organ on the womb, formed during pregnancy to support the development and growth of the foetus.
Podiatrist/Podiatry	A podiatrist is a person with specialised training in diagnosing and treating diseases of the feet. He is certified to perform minor surgeries to the foot, the scope of which depends on the training accreditation.
Polycystic ovarian syndrome	This is a condition affecting females, characterised typically, but not invariably, by obesity, presence of cysts in the ovaries, menstrual irregularities and subfertility or infertility.
Polyunsaturated fats (fatty acids)	Fats in which the fatty acids have more than one double bond (between carbon units). They occur predominantly in vegetable and seed oils, and some marine fish.
Pre-diabetes	A stage defined by specific blood glucose levels that are not normal and yet do not fulfil the diagnostic criteria of diabetes, associated with an increased risk of cardiovascular disease.
Pre-eclampsia	A complication of pregnancy characterised by high blood pressure, water retension and/or presence of protein in the urine. When coma or convulsions are also present, it is called 'eclampsia'.
Prohormone	The precursor molecule of a hormone, or any substance that can be converted into a hormone.
Proteins	Complex organic compounds consisting of carbon, hydrogen, oxygen, nitrogen and usually also sulphur, present in the amino acids which are the component units of proteins. Proteins are found abundantly in animal and fish products and in some plant products. Their role includes growth and development, cellular chemical reactions, transport and storage of other substances, mechanical support of tissues, immunity and hormone production.
Reflexology	The practice of massaging, squeezing, or pushing on parts of the feet to produce beneficial effects on other parts of the body, or to improve general health.
Retina	The innermost layer of the eyeball that receives light which is then transmitted to the brain to form images. This retina layer itself comprises an inner sublayer called the *pars nervosa* (nerve cells) and an outer sublayer called the *pars pigmentosa*.

Retinal detachment	The separation of the *pars nervosa* from the *pas pigmentosa* of the retina (see Retina).
Retinopathy	Disease of the retina.
Saturated fats (fatty acids)	Fats in which the fatty acids do not have any double bonds (between carbon units). They occur predominantly in animal fats and tropical oils.
Septicaemia	Generalised illness due to the presence of microorganisms and/or their toxins in the blood. Commonly described as blood poisoning.
SBGM	Self blood glucose monitoring.
SMBG	Self-monitoring of blood glucose or self-monitored blood glucose.
Sorbitol	A form of sugar alcohol after glucose is biochemically reduced. It is found naturally in a variety of fruits.
Stem cells	An early form of cells that have the potential to reproduce and differentiate into specialised tissues and organs.
Stomatitis	Inflammation of the oral mucosa.
Sugar	Technically, sugar is any of a class of sweet, water-soluble, crystallizable carbohydrate, and is the primary source of energy in animals. Although glucose is only one form of sugar, in this book sugar is used synonymously as glucose unless otherwise stated or implied in the text.
Sulphonylureas	A class of diabetes medication which stimulates the production and release of insulin.
Transfection	Artificial infection of animal, human or bacterial cells by uptake of genetic material from virus resulting in production of mature virus. Used in the context of gene therapy, it refers to the introduction of genetic material into host cells using a carrier or vector.
Triglyceride	Also known as neutral fat, it is a compound of glycerol and fatty acids, produced from carbohydrates for storage in animal adipose tissues.
Vitrectomy	Surgery to removed damaged or diseased vitreous (see definition below).
Vitreous haemorrhage	Bleeding into the vitreous (see definition in this Glossary).
Vitreous humour or body	A glasslike material or tissue in the eyeball in the space behind the eye lens. Sometimes shortened to 'vitreous'.

WEBSITES

American Diabetes Association
http://www.diabetes.org/about-diabetes.jsp

Centres for Disease Control and Prevention
http://www.cdc.gov/diabetes

Changi General Hospital
http://www.cgh.com.sg/library/diabetes_index.asp

Diabetes Mall
http://www.diabetesnet.com/diabetes_information/

Diabetic Society of Singapore (DSS)
http://www.diabetes.org.sg/resources.html

Diabetes UK
http://www.diabetes.org.uk

Health Promotion Board (Ministry of Health, Singapore)
http://www.hpb.gov.sg (check under 'Health A–Z' and 'Diabetes Mellitus')

International Diabetes Federation
http://www.idf.org/home/index.cfm?node=4

Singapore General Hospital
http://www.sgh.com.sg/ForPatientsnVisitors/PatientEducation/HealthGlossary/DiabetesMel

TOUCH Diabetes Support
http://www.diabetessupport.org.sg

SUPPORT GROUPS

1. Diabetic Society of Singapore (DSS)

   DSS Headquarters
   Blk 141 Bedok Reservoir Road
   #01-1529
   Singapore 470141
   Tel: (65) 6842 3382

   DSS Satellite Centres
   Hong Kah Diabetes Education and Care Centre (DSS)
   Blk 528 Jurong West St 52
   #01-353
   Singapore 640528
   Tel: (65) 6564 9818, (65) 6564 9819
   Fax: (65) 6564 9861

   Central Singapore Diabetes Education and Care Centre (DSS)
   Blk 22 Boon Keng Road
   #01-15
   Singapore 330022
   Tel: (65) 6398 0282
   Fax: (65) 6398 0275

2. TOUCH Diabetes Support
   Blk 149 Lorong 1 Toa Payoh
   #01-943
   Singapore 310149
   Tel: (65) 6252 2861
   Fax: (65) 6252 9695

REFERENCES

Preface
1. Miller LV, and Goldstein J. 1972. More efficient care of diabetic patients in a Los Angeles county hospital setting. *New England Journal of Medicine* 286: 1388

Chapter 1
1. American Diabetes Association 2010. Diagnosis and Classification of Diabetes Mellitus. *Diabetes Care* January 2010 33:S62-S69

Chapter 2
1. Diabetes Control and Complications Trial (DCCT) Research Group. 1993. The effect of intensive treatment of diabetes on the development and progression of long-term complications in insulin-dependent diabetes mellitus. *New England Journal of Medicine* 329:977–986
2. UK Prospective Diabetes Study (UKPDS) Group. 1998. Intensive blood-glucose control with sulphonylureas or insulin compared with conventional treatment and risk of complications in patients with type 2 diabetes. (UKPDS 33). *The Lancet* 352:837–853
3. The Diabetes Control and Complications Trial/Epidemiology of Diabetes Interventions and Complications (DCCT/EDIC) Study Research Group. 2005. Intensive diabetes treatment and cardiovascular disease in patients with type 1 diabetes. *New England Journal of Medicine* 353:2643–2653

Chapter 3 (Part 1)
1. Ministry Of Health website: *http://www.hpb.gov.sg/* (check under 'Health A–Z' and 'Diabetes Mellitus')

Chapter 3 (Part 2)
1. Shankar P, Choy MY, Cheong M, et al. 2005. Comparative plasma glucose and triglyceride responses in patients with diabetes mellitus to Diabetrim® instant noodles and a locally available popular instant noodles (Abstract). Presented at the 6th International Diabetes Federation (Western Pacific Region) Congress, 22–26 October 2005, Bangkok, Thailand
2. Ministry Of Health website: *http://www.hpb.gov.sg/* (check under 'Health A–Z' and 'Diabetes Mellitus')

Chapter 3 (Part 4)
1. Nissen SE and Wolski K. 14 June 2007. Effect of Rosiglitazone on the Risk of Myocardial Infarction and Death from Cardiovascular Causes. *New England Journal of Medicine* 356(24):2457–2471

2. HSA (Health Science Authority) Adverse Drug Reaction News, March 2008 Vol. 10 No. 1, 2–3

Chapter 4

1. Singapore Health Promotion Board. Monitor Your Blood Glucose At Home. *http://hpb.gov.sg/chronicdisease/diabetes/control_monitor.htm*
2. Ministry Of Health Clinical Practice Guidelines 3/2006. Diabetes Mellitus. *http://www.moh.gov.sg/mohcorp/publications.aspx/id=16462*
3. American Diabetes Association. 2008. Standards of Medical Care in Diabetes, 2008. *Diabetes Care* 31 (Suppl. 1): S12–S54. *http://care.diabetesjournals.org/cgi/content/full/31/Supplement_1/S12/T9*

Chapter 10

1. Monira Al-Arouj, Radhia Bouguerra, Buse, J., et al. 2005. Recommendations for Management of Diabetes During Ramadan. *Diabetes Care* 28:2305–2311

Chapter 12

1. American Diabetes Association. 2008. Standards of medical care in diabetes, 2008. Position Statement. *Diabetes Care* 31 (Suppl. 1): S12-54
2. Menato G, Bo S, and Signorile A, et al. 2008. Current Management of Gestational Diabetes Mellitus. *Expert Review of Obstetrics & Gynecology* 3(1):73–91
3. American Diabetes Association 2010. Diagnosis and Classification of Diabetes Mellitus. *Diabetes Care* January 2010 33:S62-S69

Chapter 15

1. American Diabetes Association. 2008. Standards of medical care in diabetes, 2008 Position Statement. *Diabetes Care* 31 (Suppl. 1):S12–S54

Chapter 17

1. Liu JP, Zhang M, Wang WY, and Grimsgaard S. 2004. Chinese herbal medicines for type 2 diabetes mellitus. *The Cochrane Collaboration.* *http://www.cochrane.org/reviews/en/ab003642.html*
2. Chang HY, Wallis M, Tiralongo E. 2007. Use of complementary and alternative medicine among people living with diabetes: literature review. *Journal of Advanced Nursing* 58(4):307–19
3. Ken Q Gu, E-Shyong Tai, Su-Chi Lim and Heok-Seng Lim. 2000. Herbal use is less reported, less consulted and found no effect for Singaporeans with diabetes. *Diabetes: A Journal of the American Diabetes Association* 49 (Suppl. 1): A387 (Abstract 1629–PO). Abstract Book of the 60th Scientific Sessions, June 9–13, 2000
4. Health Science Authority press release (16 May 2008): HSA Updates on Fatalities and Serious Adverse Reactions Associated With the Use of Illegal Health Products—Power 1 Walnut. *http://www.hsa.gov.sg/publish/etc/medialib/hsa_library/corporate/ pr20072009* Par.62900.File.tmp/MediaRelease-HSAUpdatesOnFatalities&A DRAssociatedWithTheUseOfHarmfulIllegalHealthPdts–16May2008.pdf
5. Ceriello A. 2003. New insights on oxidative stress and diabetic complications may lead to a "causal" antioxidant therapy. *Diabetes Care.* 26:1589-1596

6.   Chertow B. 2004. Advances in diabetes for the millennium: vitamins and oxidant stress in diabetes and its complications. *MedGenMed*. 6(3 Suppl):4

7.   Lee A. Witters. 2001. The blooming of the French lilac. *Journal of Clinical Investigations*. 108(8): 1105–1107

8.   Shane-McWhorter L. 2001. Biological complementary therapies: A focus on botanical products in diabetes. *Diabetes Spectrum* 14:199-208

9.   Shanmugasundaram ERB, Rajeswari G, Baskaran K, et al. 1990. Use of Gymnema sylvestre leaf extract in the control of blood glucose in insulin-dependent diabetes mellitus. *Journal of Ethnopharmacology* 30(3):281–294

10. Baskaran K, Kizar B, Ahamath K, et al. 1990. Antidiabetic effect of a leaf extract from Gymnema sylvestre in non-insulin-dependent diabetes mellitus patients. *Journal of Ethnopharmacology* 30(3):295–306

11. Althuis MD, Jordan NE, Ludington EA, Wittes JT. 2002. Glucose and insulin responses to dietary chromium supplements: a meta-analysis. *American Journal of Clinical Nutrition*. 76(1):148–55

12. Sotaniemi EA, Haapakoski E, Rautio A. 1995. Ginseng therapy in non-insulin dependent diabetic patients. *Diabetes Care* 18:1373–1375

13. Vogler BK, Pittler MH, Ernst E. 1999. The efficacy of ginseng. A systematic review of randomised clinical trials. *European Journal of Clinical Pharmacolology*. 1999 October; 55(8):567–75

14. Andersen T, Fogh J. 2001. Weight loss and delayed gastric emptying following a South American herbal preparation in overweight patients. *Journal of Human Nutrition and Diet* 14(3):243–50

15. Opala T, Rzymski P, Pischel I, et al. 2006. Efficacy of 12 weeks supplementation of a botanical extract-based weight loss formula on body weight, body composition and blood chemistry in healthy, overweight subjects—a randomized double-blind placebo-controlled clinical trial. *European Journal of Medical Research* 11(8):343–50

16. Basch E, Gabardi S, Ulbricht C. 2003. Bitter melon (Momordica charantia): a review of efficacy and safety. *American Journal of Health-System Pharmacy*. 60(4):356-9

17. Dans AM, Villarruz MV, Jimeno CA, et al. 2007. The effect of Momordica charantia capsule preparation on glycemic control in type 2 diabetes mellitus needs further studies. *Journal of Clinical Epidemiology*. 60(6):554–9

18. Alam Khan, Mahpara Safdar, Mohammad Muzaffar Ali Khan, et al. 2003. Cinnamon Improves Glucose and Lipids of People With Type 2 Diabetes. *Diabetes Care* 26:3215–3218

19. Mang B, Wolters M, Schmitt B, et al. 2006. Effects of a cinnamon extract on plasma glucose, HbA, and serum lipids in diabetes mellitus type 2. *European Journal of Clinical Investigations* 36(5):340–4

20. Suppapitiporn S, Kanpaksi N, Suppapitiporn S. 2006 The effect of cinnamon cassia powder in type 2 diabetes mellitus. *Journal of Medical Association of Thailand*. 89 Suppl 3:S200–5

21. Baker WL, Gutierrez-Williams G, White CM, et al. 2008. Effect of Cinnamon on Glucose Control and Lipid Parameters. *Diabetes Care*. 31(1):41–43

22. Velussi M, Cernigoi AM, De Monte A, et al. 1997. Long-term (12 months) treatment with an anti-oxidant drug (silymarin) is effective on hyperinsulinemia, exogenous insulin need and malondialdehyde levels in cirrhotic diabetic patients. *Journal of Hepatology* 26:871–879

23. Huseini HF, Larijani B, Heshmat R, et al. 2006. Efficacy of Silybum marianum (L.) Gaertn. (silymarin) in the treatment of type II diabetes: a

randomized, double-blind, placebo-controlled, clinical trial. *Phytotherapy Research* 20(12):1036–9

24. Hussain SA.2007. Silymarin as an adjunct to glibenclamide therapy improves long-term and postprandial glycemic control and body mass index in type 2 diabetes. *Journal of Medicinal Food.* 10(3):543–7

25. Gupta A, Gupta R, Lal B. 2001. Effect of Trigonella foenum-graecum (fenugreek) seeds on glycaemic control and insulin resistance in type 2 diabetes mellitus: a double-blind placebo controlled study. *Journal of the Association of Physicians of India.* 49:1057–61

26. Lu FR, Shen L, Qin Y, et al. 008.Clinical observation on trigonella foenum-graecum L. total saponins in combination with sulfonylureas in the treatment of type 2 diabetes mellitus. *Chinese Journal of Integrative Medicine.* 14(1):56–60

27. Hannan JM, Ali L, Rokeya B, et al. 2007. Soluble dietary fibre fraction of Trigonella foenum-graecum (fenugreek) seed improves glucose homeostasis in animal models of type 1 and type 2 diabetes by delaying carbohydrate digestion and absorption, and enhancing insulin action. *British Journal of Nutrition.* 97(3):514-21

28. Smith DM, Pickering RM, Lewith GT. 2008. A systematic review of vanadium oral supplements for glycaemic control in type 2 diabetes mellitus. *Quarterly Journal of Medicine* 101(5):351-8

29. Stevinson C, Pittler MH, Ernst E. 2000. Garlic for treating hypercholesterolemia. A meta-analysis of randomized clinical trials. *Annals of Internal Medicine* 420-9

30. Ackermann RT, Mulrow CD, Ramirez G, et al. 2001. Garlic shows promise for improving some cardiovascular risk factors. *Archives of Internal Medicine* 161(20):2505-6

31. Ashraf R, Aamir K, Shaikh AR, Ahmed T. 2005. Effects of garlic on dyslipidemia in patients with type 2 diabetes mellitus. *Journal of Ayub Medical College, Abbottabad* 17(3):60-4

32. Sobenin IA, Nedosugova LV, Filatova LV, et al. 2008. Metabolic effects of time-released garlic powder tablets in type 2 diabetes mellitus: the results of double-blind placebo-controlled study. *Acta Diabetologia* 45(1):1-6

33. Silagy CA, Neil HA. 1994: A meta-analysis of the effect of garlic on blood pressure. *Journal of Hypertension* 12:463–468, 1994

34. Foster TS. 2007. Efficacy and safety of alpha-lipoic acid supplementation in the treatment of symptomatic diabetic neuropathy. *Diabetes Education* 33(1):111–7

Chapter 18 (Part 2)

1. Foster GD, Wyatt HR, Hill JO, et al. 2003 A randomized trial of a low-carbohydrate diet for obesity. *New England Journal of Medicine* 348:2082–2090

2. Stern L, Iqbal N, Seshadri, et al. 2004. The effects of low-carbohydrate versus conventional weight loss diets in severely obese adults: one-year follow-up of a randomized trial. *Annals of Internal Medicine* 140:778–785

3. Nordmann AJ, Nordmann A, Briel M, et al. 2006. Effects of low-carbohydrate vs low-fat diets on weight loss and cardiovascular risk factors: a meta-analysis of randomized controlled trials. *Archives of Internal Medicine* 166:285–293

Chapter 19

1. Tura A, Maran A, and Pacini G. July 2007. Non-invasive glucose monitoring: Assessment of technologies and devices according to quantitative criteria. *Diabetes Research and Clinical Practice* (Vol 77, Issue 1):16–40

2. Bloomgarden ZT 6–10 June 2008. Novel Treatments for Hyperglycemia. ADA (American Diabetes Association) 2008: Emerging Treatments for Hyperglycemia. *Medscape Diabetes & Endocrinology.* *http://www.medscape.com/viewarticle/578177*

3. Braverman LE, DeFronzo RA, Fonseca VA, et al. 19 September 2008. Glycemic control for the kidney, by the kidney: Exploring the role of SGLT2 inhibition in Type 2 diabetes mellitus. *Medscape Diabetes & Endocrinology.* *http://www.medscape.com/viewprogram/17081*

4. *International Pancreas Transplant Registry*, University of Minnesota. 2004 Annual Report. *http://www.iptr.umn.edu/IPTR/annual_reports/2004_annual_report.html*

ABOUT THE AUTHORS

DR LIM HEOK SENG studied medicine at the University of Singapore (the predecessor of the National University of Singapore). He did postgraduate clinical attachments in endocrinology and diabetes at St. Thomas' Hospital and the Diabetes Clinic in King's College Hospital, London, and received his certification in endocrinology from the Academy of Medicine, Singapore, in 1990.

A former vice president of the Diabetic Society of Singapore, he was the editor of the Society's previous newsletter (*DM Life*) for five years and also contributed a chapter on "Management of Type 2 Diabetes Mellitus" in *Clinical Approach to Medicine*, a publication (2005) of the Singapore General Hospital. He was a member on SingHealth's Diabetes Health Management Advisory Board from 2002 to 2003.

Dr Lim's more recent appointments were as Director of the Diabetes Centre, Singapore General Hospital, from 1995 to 2001, and Director of the Diabetes Centre, Changi General Hospital, from 2002 to 2008, during which period he also served in CGH's Pharmaceutical and Therapeutics Committee as its vice chairman. He was, from 1998 to 2008, a member of the Ministry of Health's Special Training Committee (Endocrinology) which oversees the curriculum of specialist endocrinology training and the selection and examination of trainees in endocrinology. He was also a committee member of the Chapter of Endocrinology, College of Physicians, Academy of Medicine, Singapore, 2005–2009.

Dr Lim's current clinical practice is in the field of diabetes and general endocrinology.

JONATHAN SEAH, Senior Pharmacist at Changi General Hospital, graduated from the National University of Singapore in 2002 with an honours degree in pharmacy. He is currently the Drug Information

Pharmacist at Changi General Hospital, providing regular updates to other healthcare professionals on advances in medication therapy. Jonathan Seah is a member of CGH's Pharmacy and Therapeutics Committee, which is involved in deciding the list of medicines available in the hospital and ensuring the safe and effective use of medications. As a member of the hospital's Patient Safety Committee, he also participates actively in enhancing medication safety and improving patient education.

MAGDALIN CHEONG is Chief Dietitian/Senior Manager of the Dietetic & Food Services Department, Changi General Hospital (CGH). She graduated as a Dietitian from the Polytechnic of North London (now University of North London), UK, and is a registered dietitian with the British Dietetic Association and an accredited dietitian with the Singapore Nutritionist and Dietetic Association. She has many years of dietetic experience in general medicine and surgery, and clinical experience both in UK (including the Royal London Hospital, Whitechappel and Whipps Cross Hospital) and Singapore hospitals (Toa Payoh Hospital and CGH). Her experience in endocrinology has enabled her to work closely with diabetic patients, in the in-patient setting as well as in the community.

As Chief Dietitian of CGH, Magdalin Cheong was instrumental in setting up the dietetic service for the Diabetes Centre as well as the Dietetic and Food Services Department. She has been involved in studies related to Type 2 Diabetes, calcium intake in the elderly, cholesterol reduction and irritable bowel syndrome and has also developed dietetic programmes for patients on therapeutic diets. Recently, together with Marshall Cavendish, she has published a book entitled *A Cookbook for Diabetics*.

TAN LI JEN is Senior Clinical Psychologist at Changi General Hospital. She holds a masters in Clinical Psychology from the University of Queensland, Australia, and has been a practising psychologist for more than 10 years. Whilst undergoing training at Ipswich General Hospital in Queensland, she provided psychological support to diabetic patients, including stress and anxiety management. She has completed advanced training in 'Motivational Interviewing', an approach which helps people to change and sustain behavioural and lifestyle habits. At CGH, Tan Li Jen works with a wide range of patients who include those struggling with depression, anxiety, post-traumatic stress disorder and parenting stress, as well as with adolescents. Tan Li Jen's clinical interests are in trauma and abuse recovery, child and family mental health, anxiety and mood disorders, and clinical health psychology.